Python Programming for Beginners

The Easiest and Quickest Way to Learn Python Coding, Programming, and Web Development in Just 7 Days (Beginner's Guide 2022 Edition)

Ike Beck

TABKE OF CONTENTS

Introduction

Thank you for investing in Computer Programming for beginners. Thank you for taking the time to learn python, the computer programming language, faster and easier.

You'll find a number of highly significant and necessary notions in this book that will help you get started with Python programming. Furthermore, you will find numerous examples that will assist you in grasping the concepts we have discussed in a more visual manner.

In the following chapters, you'll find a brief overview of how programming languages evolved, who invented Python, and who uses Python today, as well as all the information you'll need to learn Python from scratch, including variables, operators, data types, functions, loops, statements, exceptions, how to create classes and modules, a chapter on Object-Oriented Programming, also known as OOP, file handling for.txt,.PDF, and.xlsx files, and much more.

We strongly advise that you study the codes here, examine them, comprehend them, and then try to create an example utilizing each one to help you remember them. Because, as you'll see, there are a plethora of commands and statements that are difficult to learn and remember if they aren't used.

There are many books on this subject available; thank you for selecting this one! We made every attempt to include as much valuable information as possible; please enjoy!

Chapter 1:
Introduction to Python

Programming can be defined as the process of planning, developing, debugging, and maintaining the source code of a computer program, or the stages involved in the generation of computer program source code.

The programming language is made up of all the rules, symbols, and phrases that are needed to create a program and, with it, provide a solution to a specific problem. Basic (1964), C++ (1983), Python (1991), Java (1995), and C# (2000) are some of the most well-known programming languages.

Programming is one of the stages in software development; it defines the structure and behavior of a program and checks whether it is working properly. Programming entails defining an algorithm, which is described as the sequence of steps and operations that a program must do in order to solve a problem. For the algorithm to work, the program must be written in a language that is compatible and correct.

Programming might be considered even easier than learning a new language because it is governed by a set of principles that are generally similar, therefore it could be considered a natural language.

To gain a better understanding of the subject of programming, we may begin by looking into the origins of programming and how all of the languages and programs we know today came to be. We could begin by saying that programming began when the first computer was created in the fifteenth century, when a machine capable of performing basic operations and square roots appeared (Gottfried Wilhelm von Leibniz), though the differential machine for calculating polynomials with the support of Lady Ada Countess (1815-1852), known as the first person to enter programming, and the differential machine for calculating polynomials with the support of Lady Ada Countess (1815-1852), known as the

It was originally designed in binary codes (bi=2), which are sequences of 0s and 1s that the computer understands directly, or machine language, which is deemed essential for the commuter to be able to interpret the information provided. Later, high-level languages arose, which used English words to give orders to obey, and which used intermediate procedures between the language and the computer, such as a compiler or an interpreter.

These programming languages have a lot simpler syntax than ours, as well as a much smaller vocabulary and set of rules. In short, programming is a sequence of phrases written in a programming language that tells the computer what tasks to execute and in what order, through a series of detailed instructions.

Interpreted languages, such as JavaScript, are computer languages in which a program called an interpreter executes the sentences while reading the text file in which they are written, which is why these programs are also known as scripts.

On the other hand, compiled languages such as Java require us to first convert the text file to a translation using a program called a compiler, and the resulting file is the one that will eventually execute on the computer.

We will focus on the Python programming language in this book, which is an interpreted language whose major and most important feature is the use of a syntax that encourages the use of understandable code. We could say that an interpreter is a form of program that executes code without the requirement for it to be compiled, which is exactly what our target language accomplishes.

What exactly is Python?

Python is a general-purpose programming language that is one of the most used nowadays. In this book, you will learn the basics of Python so that you may get started with it. Because it has no stated purpose, this language allows you to construct a large and diverse range of applications.

Python's Origins

Guido Van Possum created this language in the early 1990s, specifically in 1989, at the Centre for Mathematics and Informatics (CWI, Netherlands), as Van Rossum himself explained in one of his interviews: " "I was looking for a hobby programming project to keep me occupied during the Christmas weeks in December 1989. My office would be closed, and all I'd have at home is my computer. I decided to develop an interpreter for a new scripting language I'd been working on recently: a Unix/c descendent. Python's name was chosen for the project since I was in a bit irreverent mood (and a great admirer of Monty Python's Flying Circus)."

It was first implemented in December 1989, and the first public version, version 0.9.0, was released in February 1990. Version 1.0 was launched in January 1994, followed by version 2.0 in October 2000, and finally version 3.0 in December 2008.

This programming language is based on the philosophy of having a syntax that favors readable code; it is a high-level language that can be extended with C or C++; it has several programming environments that allow users to edit programs, interact with the interpreter, develop projects, and debug, among other things; and it is currently supported by a large community that facilitates learning and produces new progress in its already known new versions.

Python is a high-level, interpreted, and multifunctional programming language that is now one of the most popular programming languages for software development. It has become a very valuable tool in the field of programming in recent years; this language is licensed as free software, under an Open Source or open-source license approved by OSI (Open System Interconnect), and thus it is a program that can be used and distributed freely, whether for personal or commercial purposes. "To promote, protect, and enhance the Python programming language, as well as to encourage and assist the establishment of a diverse and multinational community of Python programmers," says the Python Software Foundation.

The primary benefit of an open and free technology is that it can be used without incurring licensing fees. One of the most popular technology revolutions in the twenty-first century is free software.

This language can be used in any context and disseminated at the user's discretion, with the ability to modify it if necessary, resulting in a quick and straightforward fundamental tool for program development.

To understand why we should learn Python, we must first grasp its primary characteristics, which is why we will begin by discussing its main traits:

- It's a multi paradigm programming language, which means we don't have to stick to a single manner of programming; instead, we can do object-oriented programming, iterative programming, and functional programming, so we're not limited to a single paradigm.

- It's a multiplatform language, which means we may use it to develop in a variety of contexts and operating systems, including Windows, Linux, and others.

- It is a very simple and minimalist language to learn, and this is one of the main reasons why most people choose Python as their first programming language, because it has the simplest syntax to learn. It is an interpreted language, which means that when executing a program, it will be able to execute itself, taking instructions one by one.

- It employs dynamic typed data, which can be stated as follows: when we establish a variable and store an initial type of data to it, the dynamic typed data means that this variable can change and store another value of another kind of data throughout the program, as we will see later.

- At the moment, we can also note that this language is ranked fourth in the TIOBE index, which ranks languages according to their current popularity, with Java in first place, C in second, C++ in third, and Python in fourth, indicating that it is a very popular and widely used language nowadays.

Now that we understand the characteristics of the program, we can distinguish why we should learn Python and how it will benefit us, as well as what we can program with it. Because Python is a general-purpose language, it can be used to program almost anything: desktop applications with graphical interfaces and databases, web applications, games, custom applications, and even as a point of sale system for you.

We'll talk about the language's development environment now. A development environment is a text editor in which we may copy all of the Python code, execute our programs, run our tests, and so on. We'll mention a few of these editors, including PyCharm, PyDev, Sublime Text 3, ATOM, VIM, and others, but we'll be using Visual Studio Code in this book.

What am I able to accomplish with Python?

Because it is a basic and easy to learn language with a high learning curve, like many modern languages, and a very clean and simple syntax, as stated above, it is a very versatile language, as we can develop desktop and web applications with it and the standard library. Python's object-oriented programming (OOP) support is excellent, and the only limit to what you can do with it is your imagination. This programming language is designed in such a way that there is always a better way to do something. This language is also used to work with artificial intelligence or robotics, although it is now most commonly used for Big Data because it can manage large amounts of data and sophisticated procedures.

In the field of video games: Because Python is an interpreted language, it is twice (or more) slower than a compiled language like Java, C++, or C#; you can create amazing games in Python using libraries like Pygame, SDL2 (Binding), and OpenGL (binding), but your game will not run as an executable made with C++, but rather as a Python script. However, you will have a fantastic language with plenty of help and documentation and relatively little lines of code.

Finally, there's the scientific field, which is where Python really shines. Python's syntax and the libraries it comes with by default make it ideal for scientific programming, and there are large libraries for mathematics and all that implies in the Python community.

What are the advantages of Python as a programming language?

We could say that we should use it because it is a very versatile and general-purpose language, which means that if your scope is not defined, you can create a huge number of applications using this language. For example, suppose your main goal is to create a web application; you can do it with Python, but tomorrow your interest will most likely be in scientific applications, which you can also do with Python. In fact, the main development area of this programming language is the scientific area; nevertheless, if you want to construct a low-level application or utilize it in hardware since it is also possible with this programming language, you can do so. That is why, because it lacks a clearly defined scope, we refer to it as a versatile language.

Today, who uses Python? This programming language is currently quite popular; also, it has a wide range of applications, ranging from data compilation and processing to computer learning, which is why many of the world's most important firms are currently using it. We'll mention a few of these businesses:

1. Google; it is a corporation that has worked with this language since its inception; in fact, one of its founders stated in an interview that "Python where we can, C++ where we must." This leads us to believe that when memory control is critical, Google uses C++. As a result, it is now one of the company's official languages, alongside C++, Java, and Go, which are the other three. It's worth noting that Guido van Rossum worked at Google from 2005 to 2012, demonstrating the importance of Python to the company.

2. Facebook; in this company, Python is also a part of this important social network, ranking third in

terms of most commonly used languages, just behind C++, for example; more than 5,000 confirmations of service and utilities, such as infrastructure management, binary distribution, hardware images, and operational automation, are handled in this company. As previously said, the ease of use of Python's libraries allows engineers to focus on brand optimization rather than maintaining a large number of codes.

3. Due to how fast it is to write and encode on Python, Spotify, one of the most important music corporations today, is a large Python operator. Spotify uses a massive volume of analysis and Luigi, a Python tool that synchronizes with Hadoop, to deliver suggestions and recommendations to all of its users.

4. Netflix; this corporation, like Spotify, relies on python to improve its server-side analyses. The majority of the engineers at this company have the option of working in any language they want, and the majority of them prefer to encode in this language.

5. Dropbox; at its client's desktop, this cloud-based storage system uses this language. Rossum joined this company in 2012 on the condition that he be allowed to work as an engineer alone, not as a leader or manager. During his time there, he contributed to create the option to share data warehouses with other Dropbox customers.

6. ILM (Industrial Light and Magic) is a special effects company formed by George Lucas in 1975 to create special effects for the Star Wars films. ILM chose Python 1.4 because it is easier to incorporate into their current infrastructure and because Python's interoperability with C+ and C++ made it simple to integrate Python into their unique lighting software.

In this way, we can see how Python is being used in an increasing number of places to wrap software components, expand graphic programs, and perform other tasks; it also has a large number of code libraries and is more sensitive in development regions.

How can I figure out the Python version to use?
There are presently two versions of Python that are incompatible with one another, which causes a lot of confusion for anyone learning to program, even if they are learning the same language. These versions are known as Python 2.x, which was introduced in 2000 and was updated until 2010, but version 3.x, which was issued in 2008 and is currently in full development of new versions and enhancements in their commands, was released in 2008.

Do these versions, however, include the same tools?
Well, there are significant differences between each version of Python, one of which is that in Python 3.x, the print phrase is treated as a function, so you must call it and put anything you want to print in parentheses. In contrast to version 2.x, which does not require parentheses to print, version 3.x does.

The key-value elements are utilized by the items and iterates methods in Python version 2.x when iterating a dictionary. This procedure is only possible in Python 3.x using the items, keys, and values methods, and utilizing the iterates method will result in an Attribute Error exception.

There's also a change in the input method, which takes data without transforming the variable type in Python 2.x. If we enter an integer variable in this version, its entry will be of the "int" type, and if we want it to be regarded as a string, we must call the function "raw input," which will convert "int" data to string.

This is a major step ahead in Python 3.x because the "raw input" method is silenced and any conversion can be done easily with the input function.

How can I install Python according to my operating system now that I know which version to use?
The Python programming language is included by default in Mac OS and Linux operating systems; all you have to do is upgrade to the latest version; however, Windows users will need to install the application because it is not included in the system.

Python should be installed on Windows.
Go to **https://www.python.org/downloads/** for more information.

Select your preferred version to install: 2.x or 3.x. The current version of Python (3.x) is always suggested for new users, as it simplifies understanding thanks to its streamlined tools. If you're utilizing recycled code, though, you should stick to the version that was written. Run the software once it has completed downloading. It is advised that you install Python using the default settings if you are a new user. You can execute the custom installation if you are a language expert.

Check that the program and its interpreter are both working properly.

Python for Mac OS can be installed or upgraded.

Python 2.7 is installed by default on OS X. If you need to upgrade to version 3.x, simply follow these instructions:

When you go to python.org/downloads on your computer, the link will automatically detect your operating system and show you the files that are compatible with your computer, allowing you to begin the download.

If you are a new user, click on the PKG file to begin the installation process.

Start the Python program by typing "Python3" to launch the updated version's interface.

Python for Linux: Installing or Upgrading

Python is installed by default in almost all Linux distributions, so it is not necessary to install it; the only difference is that the vast majority of distributions come with Python 2.x, rather than Python 3.x, as it should be, especially considering that most modern applications require or recommend version 3.x to compile.
Simply follow these procedures to upgrade Python:

Because the Linux Operating System is bundled with the program, but its version may vary, check the Python version you have.

Type "sudoapt-get install Python" on the Linux terminal.

Then type "sudo yum install Python" in the same terminal.

Type "pacman-S python" to log in as the root user.

Finally, start the application and verify that it functions properly before you begin programming.

Python is an excellent language to learn.
After you've downloaded Python, you'll need a code editor to help you interpret and write computer code. There is a wide range of editors available; this is

dependent on the user's preferences and amount of programming experience, as it will be your ally while programming.

Visual Studio Code is one of the most well-known editors. It's a multi-platform source code editor with a dark interface and a user interface that's been optimized. This editor includes a lot of features, including the ability to amend our code in real time as its being compiled. You don't require a full IDE, and the themes it provides allow you to customize the look of your interface.
Python, PHP, Java, C++, Ruby, Go, C, SQL, JavaScript, Batch, and Objective-C are among the languages supported by Visual Studio Code.

Sublime Text: This is a multiplatform editor with a dark design that allows you to work on a wide range of documents in several tabs and includes a full-screen mode, allowing you to maximize your computer's visual area. This contains a panel that allows you to quickly and simply navigate the code. Sublime Text can comprehend a wide range of programming languages (including Python, CSS, C++, HTML, Mat lab, R, SQL, C, Php) and includes auto save. Another feature of this editor is that it allows you to launch Python files with just a keyboard shortcut (Ctrl+B).

Geany: This is a multiplatform code editor for the Linux operating system that is suitable for application and even program development for this operating system, as well as being able to run on Windows, Mac OS, and any other system that supports the GTK library. This editor is also known for being quick and light, as well as being entirely independent and supporting languages like HTML, C++, JAVA, PHP, PYTHON, and C.

Wing is a paid Python integrated development environment that is owned by the firm Wingware. It was designed with professional developers in mind. It comes with a comprehensive range of tools and capabilities for Python programming, is compatible with Windows, OS X, and Linux, and supports Python 3.x. Wing comes in three different versions: a free basic version, a personal edition, and a professional edition, all of which are extremely powerful when writing a program.

Komodo Edit is a free, open-source editor for dynamic languages such as Python, JavaScript, HTML, CSS, Perl, and Node JS. Komodo is one of the most popular code editors for applications today, and it also comes with a premium package that contains a lot of essential features such as real-time code editing and collaboration, database exploration, and bug removal. It is mostly aimed towards small-scale project developers.

Ninja IDE: This is a development text editor that will only allow us to construct Python projects and run them at the same time in order to catch any mistakes that may occur.

Python's Keywords: It is commonly known that every programming language has a set of words and commands that are reserved and can only be used for the purpose for which they were created. In Python, there is also a set of terms known as reserved words or keywords, which are nothing more than a collection of words in which each element has a unique meaning and is an essential aspect of the language's syntax for the right development of code.

These words must be written exactly as shown in the table below, which includes some of the language's reserved words. Because Python does not discriminate between upper and lower case, or as it is properly known: case sensitive, if this is not done, the program will not be able to recognize them and will throw a Name Error exception.

If we type false, the Python interpreter won't recognize that we're talking about the false operator and will throw an error because it's not defined.

The table below shows the list of keywords for Python 3.x (the version we'll be working with in the subsequent applications), which have defined about 33 reserved words; these are the same ones that make up the syntax of this programming language.
There are a few terms in this group that are regarded"

"and"	"def"	"finally"	"in"	"or"	"while"
"as"	"del"	"for"	"is"	"pass"	"with"
"assert"	"elif"	"from"	"lambda"	"raise"	"yield"
"break"	"else"	"global"	"None"	"return"	
"class"	"except"	"if"	"nonlocal"	"True"	
"continue"	"False"	"import"	"not"	"try"	

Crucial "; they are likely to be the ones we use the most, and we'll go over them in detail in the following chapters.

True and False: These are expressions whose values are thrown to us by the program as a result of logical expressions being evaluated.

And & or: These are the expressions we use as connectors for logical expressions (True & False) so that we can create much more complex expressions.

If, elif, and else: These expressions are used to construct conditional statements in order to make decisions within the same program.

These phrases are used to create loops, or more technically, repetitive blocks.

Def. and return: These expressions contain instructions that we will use to define our own functions. To put it another way, these phrases constitute a set of instructions that will be in charge of completing a specific task as specified.

Import & from: These expressions are used to add extra functionality to a program.

If you're using Python 2.x code or just want to get started, you'll notice that, unlike Python 3.x, this version only has 31 reserved terms or keywords.

"and"	"def"	"finally"	"in"	"print"	"yield"
"as"	"del"	"for"	"is"	"raise"	
"assert"	"elif"	"from"	"lambda"	"return"	
"break"	"else"	"global"	"not"	"try"	
"class"	"except"	"if"	"or"	"while"	
"continue"	"exec"	"import"	"pass"	"with"	

What are the changes between Python 2.x and Python 3.x in terms of keywords?

Below, we'll go over some of the key changes that aren't immediately apparent:

The terms "True," "False," and "None" are used in Python 3.x.
The terms "exec" and "print," which were keywords in Python 2.x, are now integrated functions in Python 3.x, with the syntax exec() and print() ().

What is the best way for me to locate these words?
There is a module called keyword module in the standard library in Python that is responsible for exporting a list named kW list. It includes all of the reserved keywords in our programming language, Python.

Another simple approach to look up these keywords is to use the help command. This is a built-in function that allows us to look up information, documentation, and acquire more information on the components of our program.

The significance of Python syntax
Now we'll discuss the most crucial topic, which will allow us to progress in our code and programming in general: The syntax; we all know Python is an interpreted programming language, but what exactly does that imply?

Tabulations, often known as indentation or spaces, are used in our Python programming language. This means that when a program is executed, it will follow an order of interpretation, which is controlled by the tab key on our keyboard, which is simply the key with arrows above Caps Lock; these tabs are used in each loop or conditional statement.

We can avoid using keys and brackets, and we can even skip using some reserved words to start and end a program that indicates a block of code, if we have proper indentation. This makes the program easier to use and operate.

Having a decent indentation also allows us to make our code look uniform, which makes it easier to understand and provides comfort to everyone who reads it, including ourselves, because we can spot an error quickly and effectively.

It's vital to note that the initial line of code should never be indented; instead, the indentation should occur after this, with four boxes of space between them.

Physical and logical lines: A Python program is made up of a set of logical lines that are connected by a number of physical lines.

But, what are physical lines, exactly?

Physical lines are the lines that are used to enumerate our code editor, or more properly, a sequence of characters that ends with the "n" character at the end of the line.

What are logical lines, exactly?

The NEWLINE token indicates the end of each line and starts another. Logical lines are those that go with Python syntactic logic components, and their end is decided by the NEWLINE token.

These physical lines can be joined using characters like parentheses (), square brackets [], and keys to make a single logical line, which is known as "implicit union of lines."

If we begin a logical line with the characters "(", "[", "", it will continue through all necessary logical lines until it reaches the closure sign ")", "[", "".

In Python, there are two sorts of statements:
Simple assertions: Statements that must be completed in a single logical line fall into this category. Consider the following scenario:

Objects to print in the program: print ()

: Raise End Search to generate exceptions (location)

Access Attributes: from sys import stdin

Access modules: import sys

Use expressions to run functions: log. write

Compound statements are those that must start with the compound statement clause and then continue with the enclosed statement on the next line. Because it will be part of the body of our code, it must be properly indented. It will always begin with a keyword and end with ":"

Sequence and iteration for, else, else, if, elif, loops while, and else are examples of compound phrases.

Make comments in the code: In Python, a remark is a collection of non-executable characters that are placed in a text line of our program. The numerical character (#) is used to denote the comment. When it comes to programming, comments can be extremely valuable for explaining each action performed in a program code to others outside the code, or even for ourselves.

Our initial program is as follows: Good day, world!
We can develop our first program once we've installed the code editor of our choice and have a basic understanding of the Python programming language syntax: Good day, world.

If you've done any programming before, you've probably wondered, "Why is "Hello World" usually the first program to enter any programming language?" Well, the simple phrase Hello World is characterized by being an exceptionally basic code, especially while executing, and can be used as a test to confirm that our software and its interpreter have been properly installed. As a result, when working with large programs, we can be confident that everything will run well.

For ease of comprehension, all examples will now be based on version 3.x.

This code will be written in the following syntax: print ("Hello World");

Using Linux to run a software

1. On your primary user's desktop, create a project directory.

2. Save the file as Helloworld.py in plain text mode.

3. Write your code's syntax.

4. Execute the command below: Home/projects/Helloworld.py.

5. When you're finished, your code should appear as shown.

To run in Windows, follow these steps:

1. In unit C: \, make a directory called projects:

2. We'll need to make a plain text file in this directory.

3. Make a code syntax.

4. Name the file Helloworld.py and save it (the name may vary according to your preference)

5. Use the MS-DOS console to run the program: C: Python27\Python C:\Projects\ Helloworld.py.   You can

do F5 from the same software, Visual Studio, or from Helloworld.py.

6. When you're finished, your code should appear on the screen as displayed.

Using Mac OS X to run a software 1. In a new browser window, click File.

2. Make a folder named after your desire where you'll save subsequent projects.

3. Within this folder, we'll need to make a new Projects folder (all programs will be stored here).

4. Select Text Edit from the Applications menu.

5. Click on Plain Text.

6. Write the program's syntax.

7. In Text Edit, select "save as" from the file menu.

8. Save the file as Helloworld.py (or whatever name you like) and place it in the previously stated folder.

9. Go to Applications, then to Utilities, and finally to Terminal.

10. Navigate to the location where you saved your program.

11. Open the folder's cd.

12. Run lbs. and the file Helloworld.py should appear on the screen.

13. Type helloworld.py into the command prompt. Once you've completed this, your code should appear as shown.

Chapter 2:
Variables

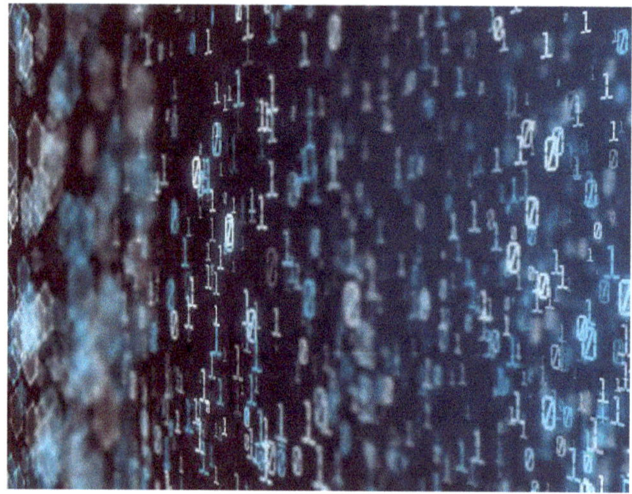

Controlling the flow of information

What exactly are flowcharts? They are tools that are used to express or develop the structure of a program or algorithm in any type of programming language.

Flow diagrams, often known as flowcharts, are a means of graphically representing an algorithm (the steps that are done in a computer) to make it easier for a person to understand.

The design of the algorithm's or program's structure can be considered the first step in the algorithm's development and preparation for the most essential step, coding.

It is recommended that when developing a software, a flowchart be created so that anyone can comprehend the algorithm's operation in a straightforward manner.

There are currently a number of software and online tools available to help in the creation of these diagrams.

Figures of importance and their significance:

	Start / end: Indicates the starting or ending of the diagram
	Input / Output of data: These are data which are assigned to the input and output variables at the beginning and ending of our code.
	Process: This is what executes the order of the operation
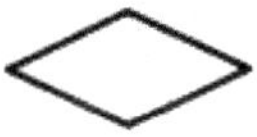	Decision: Indicates a position in the flowchart, this is used for logical expressions. In this case, the sequence is going to split in two cases, a positive and a negative one. This is also used to apply conditionals
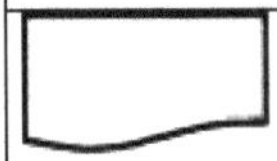	Document: This is used generally to make a document
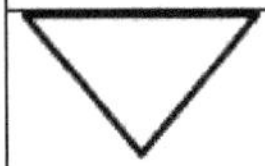	Inspection: This is used for some cases where an inspection is required.
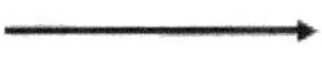	Flowline: This is used to indicate the direction of the diagram

For example:

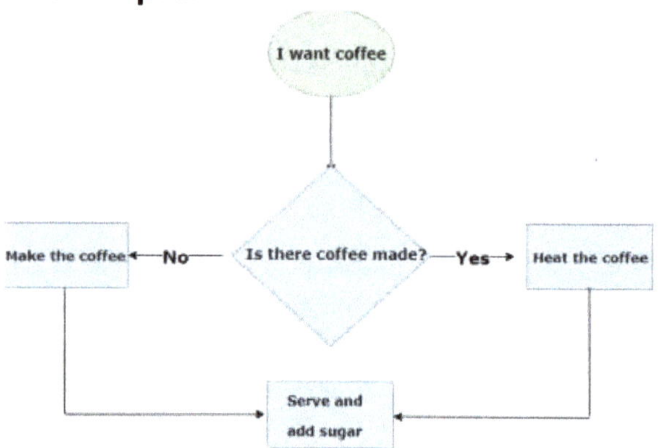

Variables

In Python, what are variables?

We have almost certainly all heard of the term "variable" in mathematics, which is defined as an unknown symbol represented by letters (x, y, z, I n) that (usually) stores a numerical value.

When we talk about variables in programming, we're referring to a space in our program's or computer's memory that may be updated and reused several times. Because they represent a box capable of storing values, these variables have a very similar form and meaning. These may store complicated words such as cities, names, passes, simple letters, and ages, unlike mathematical variables.

A variable in Python can be thought of as a "label" for the data information stored in a box, and these data can be thought of as objects. Python may also discriminate between upper and lower case letters (this is known as case sensitive), which means that calling a variable Song and calling a variable called song are not the same thing.

We must remember that because Python is an object-oriented programming language, our applications' data structures will be built on these as well. As a result, the labels we assign to variables must match the names of the instructions or else an error will occur.

In Python, declare variables. Python has the advantage of being a dynamic programming language, which means that we don't have to define the type of data we'll be working with because the interpreter can figure it out. In contrast to C++, where declaring a variable requires specifying the type of data with which the variable will be kept in memory so that the compiler can interpret it.

Consider the following scenario:

```
variable.py  ●

       ▷  variable.py
    1      variable name= value
    2
    3
    4
```

As we can see, Python assigns values to variables using the symbol "="; once this is done, the variable begins with this value, as there is no way to declare a variable without an initial value.

```
variable.py  ●

▷  ...          ▷  variable.py ▷ ...
    1     X= 2
    2     X= 4
    3
    4
    5
```

This example shows the declaration of two variables with the same name but distinct values; this is perfectly allowed because one variable is written in tiny characters while the other is written in capital letters.

It's vital to remember that in Python, certain operations aren't allowed across types (classes) that aren't compatible, so when data is identified, it becomes an inherited object of the type of data to which it belongs.

In order to declare a variable, it must be written from left to right; otherwise, a syntax error will occur.

```
variable.py

    variable.py
1   2 = X
2   4 = X
3
4   SyntaxError: can't assign to literal
```

Variable names must always begin with a letter or an underscore (the rest of the name can contain letters, numbers, and underscores).

```
variable.py

    variable.py
1   X= 2 # Valid #
2   _X= 4 #Valid#
3
4   2x = 4 #Error, starts with numeral data #

    SyntaxError: invalid syntax

    !x - False # Error, starts with symbol #
    SyntaxError: invalid syntax
```

On the same line, you can assign multiple values to multiple variables as long as the left and right arguments have the same number of arguments.

Data Types:

- Integer data in Python may identify integers of any type, including decimal, binary, hexadecimal, and octal.

There are two ways to declare an integer variable: The variable name is preceded by an int as follows:

The other method is to just write the name of the variable to be declared, which is the most usual.

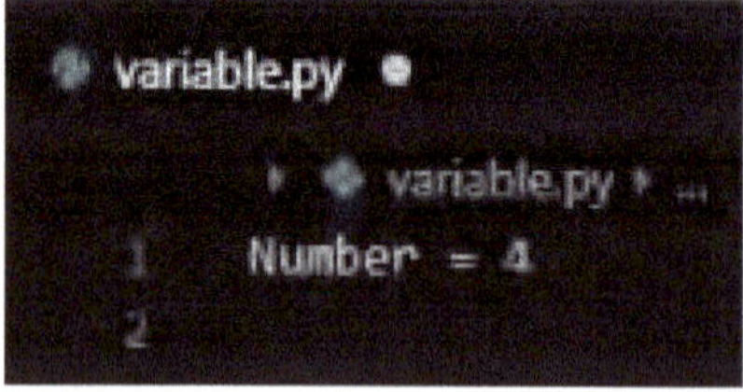

- Float: Float data is responsible for covering the entire range of real values, such as 3.14, 21, and -85.6. When we conduct an operation on float type data, we will not always get an exact value; in many cases, we will get an estimate, and its declaration is quite similar to that of integer type variables.

```
variable.py ●
        ◆ variable.py
1       Number = 4.6
2
```

- Complex: The data of the complex type relate to a sequence of operations with complex numbers, which are expressed as float data split by the operand symbol, with the first number presenting to the real number and its imaginary component being recognized by a letter j. When declaring a variable of the complex type, you must do so in the following manner:

```
variable.py ●
            ◆ variable.py ▸ ...
1       vari = complex(4+14j)
2       print(vari)
3
```

- String: A series or string of characters enclosed in apostrophes or quotation marks is referred to as string data.

String types:
\": double quotation mark.
\': single quotation mark.
\n: Line break.
\t: Tab horizontally.

Example:

```
variable.py
    variable.py ▸ ...
1   string= "Hello world"
2   string2= "This is my String example"
3   print(string)
4   print(string2)
```

- Bool: Boolean data is made up of just two (2) digits that are used to evaluate logical expressions. This is critical for future chapters since it allows us to comprehend conditionals and cycles.

A logical expression's numerical value will be 1 if it is true.

A logical expression's numerical value will be 0 if it is false.

- Lists: Data of the list type allows the software to store items of any data type, as well as the ability to have repeated items. Curly brackets are used to write these.

```
variable.py
    variable.py ▸ ...
1   a = 2
2   b = 4
3   string = "Hello people"
4   bool= True
5
6   list=[a, b, string, bool, 3, False, "good luck"]
7
8   print(list)
```

- Tuples: Tuples type data can hold several items; this type of data is similar to lists, but it differs in the following ways: Tuples are defined with a parenthesis (), unlike lists, which are declared with square brackets []; they are immutable when declared, unlike lists, which can be altered; and finally, because they are immutable, their data search is considerably more effective than that of a list.

The following is his statement:

```
variable.py

        variable.py  ...
1    a = 2
2    b = 4
3    string = "Tuple"
4    bool = True
5
6    Tup=(a, b, string, bool)
7
8    print(Tup)
```

- Set: In Python, this form of data is built on a data structure that can include several components in an undefined order. Sets can add, remove, and iterate set items, as well as execute standard operations like differentiation, verifying if an element belongs to the set, and intersecting.

We only need to name the function set to define a set (). It will return a compound of the elements if it contains a list, a tuple, or a string. Example:

```
variable.py  x

        variable.py  ...
1    A = {5, 3, 2}
2    A = set('PYTHON')
3    print(A)
```

- Dictionary data is defined as a structure with specific features that allow us to store any numeric value, list, string, or even functions. We can use dictionaries to identify each element using a key.

When working with dictionaries, it's vital to remember that the 'keys' can't be repeated data, and the keys can't be accessed by their related value. It's also crucial to note that these don't have to be in any particular order, and that the keys guide this type of data.

To define a dictionary, we encapsulate the list of values to be inserted in curly brackets. Each key pair is separated by commas, and the key is separated from the value by a colon. Consider the following scenario:

```python
user = {'name' : 'John', 'Age' : 20, 'Knowledge': ['Python progamming',"C++ programming",'JavaScript']}

print (user['name'])
print (user['Age'])
print (user['Knowledge'])
```

This will be printed:

```
John
20
['Python progamming', 'C++ programming', 'JavaScript']
```

We can see that we've generated the dictionary, and the program also displays that we've accessed each key individually.

Dictionary methods:

Get: As an argument, this method accepts a key and returns its value. If no value is found, it returns an object of type none. Consider the following scenario:

```python
user={'name' : 'John', 'age' : 20, 'knowledge': ['Python programming','C++ programming','JavaScript'] }
print(user.get('name'))
```

In this situation, it will return the name value, which is John in this example.

Item: This method is responsible for returning a list of tuples, each of which is made up of two items, the first of which is the key and the second of which is the value. Consider the following scenario:

```python
user={'name' : 'John', 'age' : 20, 'knowledge': ['Python programming','C++ programming','JavaScript'] }
print(user.items())
```

Keys () is a method that solely returns our dictionary's keys. Example:

```python
user={'name' : 'John', 'age' : 20, 'knowledge': ['Python programming','C++ programming','JavaScript'] }
print(user.keys())
```

Values: This function merely returns the values from our dictionary for their corresponding keys.

```
variable.py ×
    variable.py ...
1   user={'name' : 'John', 'age' : 20, 'knowledge': ['Python programming','C++ programming','JavaScript'] }
2   print(user.values())
```

Clear: This approach removes all of the elements from our dictionary, leaving it empty. Consider the following scenario:

```
variable.py ×
    variable.py ...
1   user={'name' : 'John', 'age' : 20, 'knowledge': ['Python programming','C++ programming','JavaScript'] }
2   print(user.clear())
```

Copy () returns a duplicate of the original dictionary. Consider the following scenario:

```
variable.py ×
    variable.py ...
1   user={'name' : 'John', 'age' : 20, 'knowledge': ['Python programming','C++ programming','JavaScript'] }
2   print(user.copy())
```

Re-declaring variables in Python:

Python has the advantage of being able to re-declare variables in a straightforward manner, from changing their value to changing the type of variable without any complexities. Consider the following scenario:

```python
a=4
print(a)
a=8
print(a)
a=True
print(a)
a= "Julia"
print(a)
```

In the last example, we can see that the variable "a" is first declared with the value 4, which is an integer, then the variable is re-declared with the value 8, indicating that the variable is still an integer, and finally, the variable is re-declared with the value True, indicating that it is now a Boolean value. Finally, we've assigned a string to the variable, which we can see as the name "Julia," indicating that the variable is now of the string type.

Concatenate String

We simply need to utilize the addition operator (+) to concatenate character strings. It's vital to notice that the area where we want to leave the space blank must be marked specifically and explicitly.

```
variable.py

    variable.py ...
1    a= "Hello world"
2    b=" this is an example"
3    c= a + b
4    print(c)
```

As seen in the previous example, the variable "a" was created with the value "Hello world," then the variable "b" was created with the value "this is an example," and finally the variable "c" was created with the value "this is an example," and this last one was in charge of carrying out the concatenation of "a" and "b."

Integer and Boolean values can also be concatenated, but this requires converting the variables to strings first. How do you go about doing this? Well, it's quite simple; we simply call the STR function. Consider the following scenario:

```
variable.py

    variable.py ...
1    string= "class of "
2    date= 2019
3    date=str(date)
4    final=string + date
5    print(final)
```

As can be seen in the example, we first generated a string variable with the value "class of," and then we created an integer type date variable with the value "2019." Then, using the function STR, we convert our variable date to a string ().

Concatenating lists is another popular example, which we perform using the method extend (), for example:

```python
lunch = ["Sanwich", "pizza", "Burger", "meat"]
snack = ["ice cream", "cookie", "brownie", "cake"]
lunch.extend(snack)
print(lunch)
```

In the preceding example, we can see that a list with some lunch alternatives was generated, followed by another list with some snack options, and lastly, the command lunch. Extend (snack) was created by concatenating list number 1 with list number 2.

Global Variables

Global variables are variables that are utilized throughout the program; once defined, they can be used as a main function or any other function.

This type of variable can be changed anywhere in the program, which may appear to be a benefit, but it may also cause confusion for the programmer and anybody else who reads the program. Another disadvantage of global variables is that they might take up more space than common variables since they cannot be deleted at the end of the function. On the other hand, this feature prevents the code from being reused, which makes Python one of the most appealing programming languages.

Working with global variables is considered bad practice in general, yet having comprehensive knowledge is never too much. After that, we'll look at how to declare a global variable.

This necessitates the usage of the global command:

```
variable.py

    variable.py ...
1    global var
2    var = 2019
3    print(var)
```

Calling or declaring a global variable is not difficult, as we saw in the previous example. We may compare it to how we declared variables; the only difference is that the variable "var" will now have a global character, allowing any function to access it easily.

Variables in the local environment
Local variables are variables that are used once and then erased from memory after the function is finished. Local variables, unlike global variables, allow us to save large numbers of lines of code, making modular programming much more agile and simple, and thus allowing code reuse, which makes Python one of the most impressive programming languages.

The main benefit of utilizing local variables in a Python program is that it makes the code easier to read and comprehend; global variables allow any issue to be rectified more quickly and efficiently. Because the number of lines of code has been reduced, it is unlikely that there will be any confusion when interpreting it.

Local variables are regarded a useful practice to utilize when programming because they are intended to produce much easier programs for people who do not have much knowledge with programming.

To help you grasp this, we'll create an example that demonstrates how to use these variables during programming.
Example: We're going to make a problem where it has to collect the following information from a person:
1. First and last names
2. Your age
3. Place of origin

```python
full_name = input("Full name: ")
age = input("Age: ")
country_origin = input("country of origin: ")
print("Full name"+full_name + "\n" + "Age"+ age + "\n"+"Country of origin" + country_origin)
```

What does it indicate that the syntax focuses more on the input () command than on anything else? This is the only function that allows for a user-program interaction. The variables "full name," "age," and "country of origin" will now have the value that the user enters into the console right now.

```
Full name: Python programmer
Age: 100
country of origin: Worldwide
```

Chapter 3:
Operators

Operators are mathematical symbols that perform a specific operation between operands, and they can take variable operands. The arguments that operators receive in order to perform their functions are known as operands. As a result, operators can be defined as special symbols capable of executing logical and arithmetic operations.

Types of operators:

- Logic operators.
- Arithmetic operators.
 - Comparison operators.
- Assignment operators.
- Special operators.

- Logical or conditional operators: These are the operators that we utilize to categorize, deny, and exclude certain of our code expressions.

1. **Operator not**: This operator is responsible for negating or returning a value that is the inverse of the Boolean value. True=False is not the case. False=False, not False=True.

2. **Operator or**: This operator evaluates the values on the right side and the values on the left side in order to return a true value if at least one condition is satisfied.

False or True = True

True or false = True

True or True = True

False or False = False

3. **Operator and**: This type of operator is in charge of determining whether the conditions between the left-hand value and the right-hand value are met correctly:

True and False = False

True and True = True

True and False = False

False and False = False

- Comparison operators: These are the operators that we use to compare (as the name implies) some values stored in the program, so that when we compile it, we can return a True/False value as a result of satisfying a condition.

1. The! = operator is in charge of determining whether these stored values are different and, depending on the outcome of the analysis, returns a True/False. E.g.

20! =20 the end result will be False.

14! = 15 True will be the outcome.

2. Operator ==: This type of operator is responsible for determining whether these values are the same for various types of data, and the result of its analysis will give us a True/False. E.g.

19 = = 19 True will be the outcome.

10 = = 5 the outcome will be False.

3. Operator >: This operator is responsible for determining whether the value entered on the left side is greater than the value entered on the right side. E.g.

30>25 True will be the outcome.

9> 28 the outcome will be False.

4. **Operator**: This type of operator determines whether the value entered on the left side is higher or lower than the value entered on the right side. E.g.

26<9 Result will be False

14 < 22 the result will be true

5. **Operator** >=: This operator is responsible for determining whether the value entered on the left side is greater than or equal to the value entered on the right side. E.g.

20> 14 the result will be true
10 > 26 the result will be False
10 >= 10 The Result will be True

6. Operator =: This type of operator is used to determine whether the value entered on the left side is less than or equal to the value entered on the right side. E.g.

20 < 11 the result will be False
16 < 25 the result will be true
15 <= 15 the result will be True

- Assignment operators: These are the sorts of operators that are used in a program to assign (as the name implies) a value to a variable; in this case, the operators will be preceded by an equals sign (=).

1. Operator Equality (=): This is the most common form of operator, and it will always be on the left side of the variable. For example, if A=10, the value of A will be 10.

2. Operator Sum - equality (+=) operator this sort of operator is in charge of adding to the left-hand variable, with the value on the right-hand side. For example, > A= 10; A += 8; A= 18

It would be the same as saying: A=10; A + 8 A=18.

3. Operator subtracts - equality (-=). This operator subtracts from the variable on the left side of the equation, with the value on the right side. E.g.

A = 10; A -= 8; A = 2

It would be the same as saying: A=10; A - 8; A= 2

4. Operator Rest - equality (%=) the remainder of the division on the left side is returned to the value on the right side by this type of operator.

>A = 10; A% = 8; A = 2

It would be the same as expressing A= 10; A percent 8; A= 2

5. Integer Operator - equality (//). The integer division of the variable on the left side by the value on the right side is calculated using this type of operator.

A = 10; A //= 8; A = 1

It would be the same as saying A= 10; A / 8; A= 1

6. Operator Product - equality (*=) is the sixth operator. This operator is in charge of multiplying the left-hand variable by the right-hand value. E.g.

> A= 10; A *= 8; A = 80

It would be the same as saying: A=10; A * 8; A=80.

7. **Equality** (/=) as a division operator. This operator is responsible for dividing the variable on the left side by the value on the right side. E.g.

>A= 10; A /= 8; A= 1, 25

It would be the same as saying A= 10; A * 8; A= 1, 25.

8. Exponent Operator - equality (**=). The exponent of the variable on the left side is calculated using this type of operator, with the value on the right side. E.g.

>A = 10; A **= 8; A = 100000000

It would be the same as saying A= 10; A **; 8 A= 100000000.

- Special Operators: These operators are frequently used in program loops to check for repeated variables and even to determine if an element is stored within another element.

1. Operator In: If an element is stored inside another, this operator will return 'True.' For example, A= [80, 40] 80 in A

Because the value 80 is located in A, the result that will be returned will be of true type.
2. Operator Is: If the values stored in the variables are the same, this type of operator will return true. E.g.

X= 80; Y= 80. X is Y

Because both variables contain the same stored value, the result will be of the True type.

3. Not in: If an element is not stored inside another element, this type of operator returns true. For example, A= [80, 40] 40 is not in A.

Because the value 40, if it is positioned in A, would return False, the result will be of the false type.

4. Operator not is: If the values stored in the variables are not equal, this type of operator will return true. E.g.

X=80; Y=40. X is not Y.

The returned result will be of the True type because both variables have different values stored in them, hence they are distinct.

- Arithmetic Operators: These are the operators used to execute basic arithmetic operations.

The sum operator (+) is a sort of operator that adds numerical values. E.g.

80 = 40 + 40

2. Subtractive operator (-): This operator subtracts values from the numerical type. E.g.

40 − 40 = 0

3. Multiplication operator (*): This operator multiplies numerical values. E.g.

1600 = 40 * 40

4. Division operator (/): This type of operator will be used to divide numerical numbers. E.g.

10 / 2 = 5

5. Exponent operator (**): This operator calculates the exponent of a recorded value between numerical data type values. E.g.

2 x 4 = 16

6. Integer Division Operator (//): This type of operator is used to calculate the integer division of a numeric data type stored value, returning only the integer part. E.g.

5 // 2 = 2

Note: When working with two integer operands, the program will presume that you want the variable to return an integer result. E.g.

Our result will be 3 if we use the formula A= 7 // 2.

Simply add at least one decimal value to either of the two operands to receive the decimals as in the first example. G = 7.0 / 2 = 3.5, for example.

7. Operator Module: The remainder of the division between the two operands is returned by this type of operator. Ex, =.

7 % 2 = 1 is the division module.

The following is the order of precedence or priority of arithmetic operators:

1. Exponent (**) is a term that refers to the number of times a
2. Module (*), Division (/), Whole Division (//), Multiplication (*), Division (//), Division (//), Division (//), Division (//), Division (percent)

The rest of the operators are grouped together in line 2, which means they all have the same order of priority, but they will be resolved by that order of precedence when they operate. Example:
When in use: 8*10/2

This indicates that the procedure should be performed as follows: 8*10= 80 / 2 = 40. Our operation yielded a score of 40.

Parentheses, on the other hand, can be used to change the order of precedence ().
Example:

When 80*(10/2) is in use

This indicates that the procedure should be performed as follows: 10/2= 5 * 4 = 20.
Let's look at two simple examples of how to use operators: one is to compute the area of a rectangle, and the other is to check whether the key is right.

The first example is the rectangle's area:

```python
b=int(input("Please enter the base: "))
h=int(input("Please enter the height: "))
print("The area is "+str(b*h))
```

The first thing we do in this example is declare the variables. The first is variable b, which is related to the base and passes through numerous stages, but we put it on one line to save space.

To clarify, the first thing we can notice is that both b and h have an input type in their declarations, indicating that it will be saved as a string. As a result, we can also see the int function, which will convert that string into an integer, allowing us to do operations on it. Do you have any idea why that is?

Because it is impossible to add two strings, because adding 1 + 1 is significantly different from adding "1" + "1," because the first is a sum of integers, and the result will be equal to 2, whereas the second is a sum of ASCII characters, and the result will be unknown. As you can see, the same thing is done with the variable h, thus b and h are two integers that the user has entered.

Because it is not feasible to concatenate a string with an integer, the function STR () is used. The next action is to print in screen the string "The area is" concatenated with the string related to the multiplication of the base and the height.

As you can see, this is a fairly simple example, but it raises an interesting question: what happens if you enter a negative value? If you enter -5 and 2, for example, the value returned will be -10, which is a significant mistake because there are no negative areas, thus it's an error in our application. Conditionals can be used to remedy the mistakes, as well as the handling of exceptions, which will account for these scenarios.

The following is a second example of key verification:

```
operators.py

1    password="12345"
2    passuser=input("Please enter the password here: ")
3    print("User "+str(password==passuser))
4
```

The first step is to declare the password variable as a string "12345," followed by the pass user variable, which is tied to the input function and will display "Please enter the password here: " on the screen, and the same will be made in pass user is a string.

Finally, if the key is correct or not, it will be printed in screen "User," which will be concatenated with the result of comparing if password is strictly equal to pass user. However, in order for this to be concatenated, it will be necessary to convert this comparison into a string, because it is necessary to delimit that when some comparison is made, the return is a string ().

Conditionals

We will base ourselves in order to be able to use the instructions with the help of logical operators, and, well, logic in general, because they will allow us to construct more sophisticated programs, because they allow us to specify conditions, such as what? Consider the following example:
If it's going to rain today, I'll wear my sweater; if it's not going to rain, I won't.

Similarly, conditionals operate because an action will be carried out if a specific circumstance is met, but if the predicted does not occur, something else will.

If, else, and elif conditionals are among the conditionals; there are other occasions where exceptions are utilized to prevent the program from collapsing.

- If a given event occurs, an action will be conducted; otherwise, nothing will happen, and the normal or expected flow will continue. This can be used for simple applications like age-based access. How? It will not allow the client to enter if he is not of legal age.

If conditional flowchart is as follows:

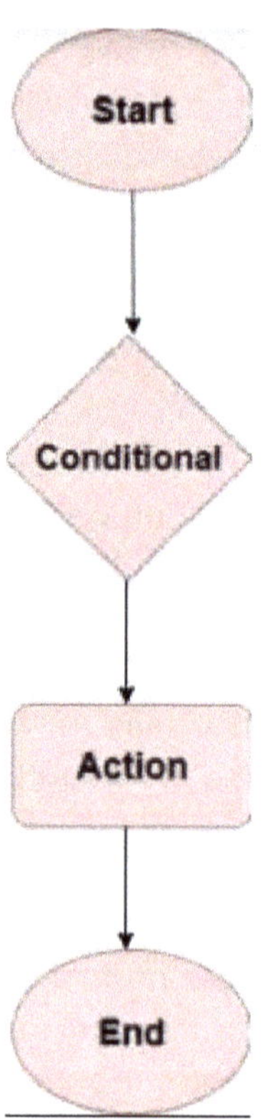

In Python, the syntax for If is as follows:

- If + condition: If the condition is met, the following commands will be executed inside this block with the required indentation.

Now, in terms of syntax, there are a few things to keep in mind when creating the if blocks:

- The if + condition is always the first line, followed by a colon (:), because it is evident that a block is being started this way.
- The instructions that will be carried out are indicated in the following lines; however, they will only be carried out if the condition is true.
- Finally, the block of instructions must have indentation because if these are not appropriately positioned, the program will not grasp what you exactly want and will either not execute what you requested or will just close the program.

This is a clearer example of the syntax, which will show whether or not a student passed an exam:

```
if.py                 ✕

1    note=input("Put your note here: ")
2    if(int(note)<5):
3        print("You didn't pass, try again")
4
```

As can be seen, a note variable was created, which is linked to the input function, and is waiting for the note that the user has obtained. This variable is of the string type.

Following that, we reach the conditional element, specifically the if, and the condition to compare is that if the user's note is less than five, a screen will print indicating that the user failed and must try again. As you can see, the int () function was used in the if condition, which is required since the note variable is a string, and a comparison of a number with a string is impossible. As a result, the type of the string variable must be changed to integer in order to make the corresponding comparison.

What if the condition isn't true? Is there anything else you can do? Well, you do, because there is another statement, the else, which is used when the if condition is false and you need to perform another action. If you want to learn more about this statement, read the following paragraphs.

- What does else + condition mean? The else condition is used when the if condition is false. This simply means that if the condition's clause is not met, the program will close immediately; to avoid this, we use the else instruction, which instructs the computer to execute a different action.

The else conditional's flowchart is as follows:

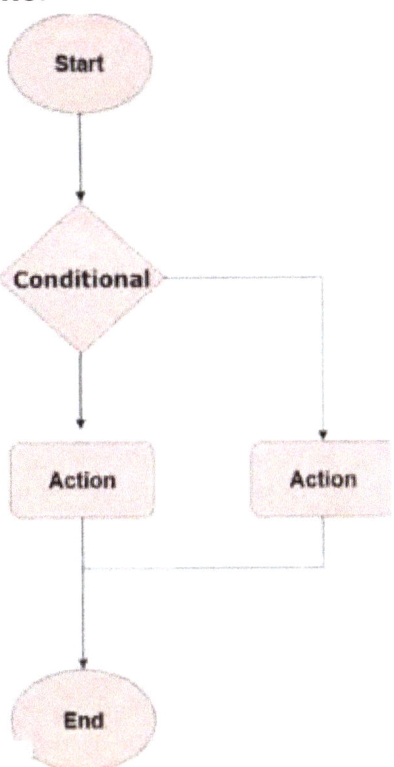

The syntax of the conditional else is fairly similar to the syntax of the conditional if, with the exception that the conditional does not have to be inserted in this case, therefore maintaining proper indentation is critical.

We will create a test program to observe the programming of the else conditional in greater detail, allowing us to clearly see the differences between conditionals.

It will be a variation on the previous program, with the goal of demonstrating how effective conditionals can be.

```python
note=input("Put your note here: ")
if(int(note)<5):
    print("You didn't pass")
else:
    print("Congatulations, you pass")
```

In this example, we can see that the note variable was created, which is an entry that the user will choose, in this case, to enter his note, so that the program can determine whether his note was sufficient to pass or not. To make it clear to the user that he must enter his note, the following string "Put your note here" will be printed on the screen, so the user understands that he must enter his note.

After that, the conditional block was added, which states that if the user's note's transformation to integer is less than five, "You didn't pass" will be written on the screen, and the program will exit since the otherwise block will not be entered because the condition is true. If the condition is false, it will be given to else, which will print the following string "Congratulations, you passed" on the screen to show users if they passed or failed the exam with their note.

As you may have seen, the usage of if and else is quite beneficial, if not essential, because it allows you to have the program produce different results rather than a single straightforward flow, which is useful because, as you might expect, programs without logical bifurcations are not generally utilized.

Another example is division, which demonstrates yet another key feature of conditionals: the denominator cannot be equal to zero, because division between zeros is not specified and would result in a mathematical error.

```python
num=input("Select the number of the numerator: ")
den=input("Select the number of the denominator: ")
if(den=="0"):
    print("Zero can't be denominator")
else:
    num=int(num)
    den=int(den)
    result=num/den
    print("The result is "+str(result))
```

Since we've already discussed the problem, we can see an example of division here.

The first step is to create the variable num, which will be tied to the division's numerator and defined next to an input function so that the user can enter the desired value. The same will be done with the den variable, which is linked to the division's denominator.

Then we'll enter the conditional block, where the condition we'll look for is that the variable den is equal to the string "0," to see if the division can be done or not. If the condition is true, the string "Zero can't be denominator" will be displayed on the screen, informing the user that the denominator he entered did not match the mathematical requirements. However, if the condition is not zero, division may be done, so we enter the else block; the first thing we do is convert the variables num and den to integers, but what is the purpose of doing so in this portion of the code? To perform mathematical operations, both num and den must be integers, but this is done in the else section as part of code optimization, because if the denominator had been zero, time would have been wasted on unnecessary instructions, because no operation would have been performed, as you already know, because division by zero is not allowed. You might think that there is no difference between doing it here and doing it elsewhere, but there is. Imagine having to do it a million times; that would result in a significant computational cost for something that will never be used. That is why it is always important to do this type of reasoning in such a way that it tries to make the program as efficient as possible.

The next step is to divide the numerator by the denominator, save the result in the result variable, and then print the result on the screen.

If you're a little bit of a programmer, or already know how to program in C or Adriano, to name a few languages, you'll be looking for the explanation of how the switch is used here in these conditional sentences, because these aren't found in Python; instead, the elif is used, and its explanation can be found below.

- Elif + condition: When there are multiple conditions, we use the elif conditional as a faster and more effective way to join an else with elif. For example, in other programming languages, the switch () conditional is frequently used to handle numerous circumstances. This is replaced in Python by elif (), which is nothing more than an additional conditional on the else to acquire numerous cases.

When you have various conditions with a variety of methods to perform, this is a frequent technique.

Now we'll look at an example to see how this works in detail, and then we'll enter the conditionals.

```python
option=input("Please enter your option, for your message: \n1)Español \n2)English \n3)Deutsch \n")
if(option=="1"):
    print("Hola")
elif(option=="2"):
    print("Hello")
elif(option=="3"):
    print("Halo")
else:
    print("Bad option")
```

The option variable has been created in the elif example, and it is related to the choice that the user wants to enter into his program. As can be seen in the code, the options are 1 for the answer to be in Spanish, 2 for the answer to be in English, and 3 for the program's answer to be in German.

When we enter the conditional block, the first thing we see is the if, which has the condition that the variable option is the same strict as the string "1," and if it is true, the string "Hello" will be displayed on the screen; if this option is not fulfilled, it will go to the first elif, which has a different condition, in this case, that the variable option is the same strict as the string "2," and if it is true, it will display the string " If no case is met, it will proceed to the else block, which means it will print a message on the console that states "Bad option."

As a result, we can see that the software has three alternatives, each of which is a message that will be displayed to the user and will say hello in a variety of languages, including Spanish, German, and English.

As we can see from the examples of conditionals, they are quite important in programming because they allow us to add a variety of alternatives to our programs and have them behave in different ways depending on the situation.

However, conditionals are not the only tools we have for special conditions; another very useful tool, which is frequently used in programming, are exceptions, which catch any errors and allow the program to run correctly. Furthermore, in the example of division by zero, you can use this tool, but not only for division by zero, but many other times as well; all you need are the tools listed below.

Handling exceptions:

When we program, we frequently encounter errors during the execution of our code. Syntax errors and exceptions are two forms of problems that we may face on our journey. Syntax errors, as we've seen, arise when we type code wrongly.

The syntax errors reported in the event of exceptions are different. What are your thoughts on this? They occur when something unexpected occurs during the execution of a program. Consider a software in which a user is asked to enter a number in order to fulfill a requirement. Consider what happens if the user types a string instead of a number while entering data. The application will display a Type Error.

When we don't properly handle exceptions, our software will crash because the interpreter won't know what to do in such a unique situation.

Returning to the previous example, we know that our program will operate as long as we enter an integer value as an input value. If we enter a string, however, the other form of mistake will be a Value Error exception.

The following are some of the most common exceptions: Name Error: The exception's nature When a program is unable to locate a global or local name, it encounters a Name Error. When the program informs us that we have been unable to locate something, it will include the incorrect name in the message.

Type Error: The exception's type. When an incorrect object is passed via the function as an argument, a Type Error occurs. When the program displays the type of error that has been supplied, it will explain how to work with the arguments correctly in detail.

The kind of exception is Value Error. Value Error happens when a function's parameter has the correct declared types but an insufficient value.

The kind of error is Not Implemented Error. When an object that supports an action is not implemented, the Not Implemented Error is thrown. When a function accepts an input parameter, these types of errors should be avoided; instead, a Type Error type exception should be used instead.

When a zero type of data is provided to the input (such as a denominator) in a division operation or module operation, a Zero Division Error type of error is thrown.

File Not Found Error: When a dictionary or file that has been requested does not exist in the program, the File Not Found Error exception type is thrown.

Exception handling: It is well known that each programming language contains a specific number of reversed words that make it easy to handle any exception that may emerge while programming. As a result, we will be able to act quickly to prevent the program from being halted.

When dealing with exceptions in Python, we employ "blocks," which are most commonly used with the try, except, and finally statements.

So, how does this function?
The following steps will be taken to raise the exception: All code that could be raised with an exception is found in the try block. (Raise is a programming phrase that refers to the act of triggering an exception.)

After that, the exception block will be located, which will be in charge of containing the exception and allowing it to be processed by sending a certain sample message.

Finally, we have the finally block, which will be used to execute an action. This will be done regardless of whether or not an exception has been raised, ensuring that the block is completed regardless of the prior conditions.

The sentence finally is always considered very useful when programming exceptions, yet its relevance is sometimes overlooked.
What is the last block? What is the purpose of it? What is the foundation for it?

Let's pretend we've developed some code in the try block that will handle a specific task and consume a big number of resources that must be released once they're no longer needed. Through the finally clause, these resources will be freed or removed, and the function will be executed regardless of whether the try block was successful in raising the exception.

Because it is impossible to divide by zero, we will use a similar scenario to demonstrate the value of working with exceptions.

```python
num=input("Please enter the numerator: ")
den=input("Please enter the denominator: ")
den= int(den)
nun=int(num)
try:
    result=num/den
    print("The result is: "+ srt(result))
except:
    print("Invalid values")
```

The first step is to declare the variable num, which is related to the input function and will be waiting for data to be entered by the user in such a way that a decimal value will be expected to be stored in num; similarly, the variable den, which is designed to be the denominator of the division, will be waiting for data to be entered in such a way that a decimal value will be expected to be stored in den.

The next step is to change the type of format of each variable; for example, the function int() is used to convert the variables num and den to integers; because they are related to an input, the same ones will be stored as a string, making arithmetic operations impossible; as a result, they are transformed to variables of type int.

Since we first entered the try block, which is in charge of attempting to perform certain actions if no exception occurs; what we mean by this is that, in this case, if den is not equal to zero, no exception should occur, so the value of the division between num and den should be stored in the variable result, and the value of it will be printed on screen.

However, if an error happens, such as an exception, it will be recorded in the exceptions and a message will be displayed on the screen stating that the entered values are invalid.

Another example that we must show is one that takes the block finally, so we can see its functionality; for this, we will continue with the divisions examples, but now we will add two exceptions: one that will appear if the values entered are not decimal, making it impossible to convert them to integers; as a result, the first exception will be triggered. The denominator will then be checked to see if it is equal to zero, and if it is, another exception will be thrown.

```python
num=input("Please enter the numerator: ")
den=input("Please enter the denominator: ")
try:
    den= int(den)
    num=int(num)
except:
    print("Error, you put a ASCII data, please try again")
    num=int(input("Please enter the numerator: "))
    den=int(input("Please enter the denominator: "))
try:
    result=num/den
    print("The result is: "+str(result))
except:
    print("Error, the den has a value equal to zero")
finally:
    print("Thanks for use this program")
```

The first thing we see, and what we should expect, is that both the variable num and the variable den are using the input() function, which is responsible for receiving the value that the user desires, in this case, the numerator and denominator values, respectively.

Then we get to the first set of instructions, which are as follows: What exactly are we attempting to accomplish in this section? The first step is to convert the strings that are both num and den to integer variables in order to continue with the appropriate mathematical operations. It is critical to accomplish this since, as you may know, it is impossible to divide a letter by another letter because it is mathematically impossible. The first is the try block, which, as its name implies, will try to accomplish something; if nothing causes an error, it will do it without difficulty; if it is not feasible, it will enter the except block, which will handle the exception. If an issue is detected, that block will go into action, attempting to correct the problem. The first thing it will do is display the error on the screen, informing you that erroneous ASCII data was put and that you should try again. Then the num variable will be re-declared as an input type variable because it will be waiting for user input, and it will be turned to an integer type variable, and the same will be done with the den variable.

The other block of exceptions will be accessed later, and the first instruction we discover there is to declare the result variable, which will be the division between the num and den, and then to display the result of the division on the screen. And, as you should know, this block will attempt to do so, but there is a chance that something may go wrong, but what could it be? The primary one is the division by zero, which is more than a programming error; it is a mathematical error. As a result, this block will not be executed, and the exception will be thrown. The same one will try to inform the user that an error has occurred; this message will inform him that the denominator has a value of zero, indicating that the division cannot be completed.

Finally, we'll reach the finally block, which will always execute an instruction regardless of what happens, regardless of whether the try or except blocks are performed. In this situation, it will print a note expressing gratitude for having utilized this application.

However, if you compare the previous and current examples, you will notice that the block finally does not do anything particularly noteworthy, but it does; the difference is that it is always done. Now, if you w
ant to see an example where the finally is used more and is more important, you will see it when working with databases, because it is always necessary to close the connection to a database, regardless of what happens, because failure to do so may result in errors that no programmer wants.

Chapter 4:
Loops

What is the definition of a loop?
A loop (or cycle) is a control structure that repeats a block of instructions while a specific condition is met; inside loops, there are also so-called endless loops, which never have their condition met. Python, like most programming languages, features a while and for clause.

1. Iterate on the items in any sequence (either a list, a string of characters, or a dictionary) in the order they appear in the sequence, using Python's for statement.

The code is referred to as "loop body" and the repetitions as "iterations."

Iteration is described as repeating a set of actions multiple times. The for loop is in responsibility of running through these operations and looking for elements that meet certain criteria while also being able to execute the provided instructions. As a result, each of these items must be alterable.

A for loop has the following syntax: loop body for variable + alterable element (list, string, range, etc.)

It is required to specify the variable in which the element's items will be kept, after which we write our sentence for with a variable that will store the things, and finally we write in which will be our iterate element.

The loop will continue to run as long as it meets the condition, so after the iteration is complete, the loop will come to an end.

Example:

```python
1   x=0
2   for x in range(4):
3       print(x)
4   print("End")
5
```

The first thing we notice is that we define the variable x, which starts at zero. This is because it will iterate, and it must begin at zero.

Then we complete the for cycle, and as you can see, the variable x is set to iterate within the range of 4 iterations. What exactly does this imply? X will iterate four times, taking the values zero, one, two, and three each time.

The next step is the block inside the for, which is a simple print, and this will display us the value that has x in each phase of the for, until it reaches the number four, at which point the cycle will automatically end.

Finally, End will be typed to indicate that the program is complete and that the cycle has been terminated.

For loops come in a variety of shapes and sizes.

1. Make for cycles with lists: You can make for cycles with lists, in which case it will iterate through each value in the list.
We'll give some instances of each of these ways of using the fore to help you grasp what we're talking about.

a. Loop "for" with list and function "range"; in this loop, list data types are presented, and a for can be created using the functions Len () and range (), which are particularly useful for printing data.

-range () is a function that, as previously said, returns a list of integers with the starting, end, and increment between one element and the next as arguments. One or two of these can alternatively be omitted, as explained below;
- Range (n); this type of function returns a list of integers that starts with 0 and ends with n-1.
- range (starting, end): this type of function returns a list of integers that fall between the beginning and the end, but do not include the latter.
- range (starting, end, step); this type of function returns a list of numbers in the same way as the previous one, only that there will be a step difference between the first and second member, and so on.

Let's look at two examples, one without and one with the range function.

1) Without the usage of range, for and lists are used:

```python
sports=['soccer', 'baseball', 'tennis', 'polo']
for x in sports:
    print(x)
print("End")
```

As you can see in the example, a list with the name sports was generated first, and it contains things such as soccer, baseball, tennis, and polo.

The for cycle was then defined, followed by the question, "What does the x variable do this time?" What it does is iterate through the sports list, giving x the values of each item in the list.

The next step is to define the for block; remember to indent since if you don't, no action will be taken because Python takes indentation extremely seriously. We define the block, which is a simple print, which prints the values of x, and as we've just explained, x will take the value of the items in the list in question.

Finally, the word "End" will be printed on the screen to indicate that the program has completed and the cycle has been properly terminated.

2) The use of for and lists, as well as range:

```python
sports=['soccer', 'baseball','tennis','polo']
for x in range(len(sports)):
    print("The sport "+str(x+1)+" is "+sports[x])
print("End")
```

We can see a difference in the example; the first is that we are using the range this time, but we will go over the code step by step to explain it and make it as clear as possible.

The first step, as we've seen, is to create a list, in this case, the same list as in the prior example, with the ramifications that this entails: the previous example's elements will be the same as the present ones.

Then we define the for, in this case, we place the range, which means that x will iterate from zero to the range of integers returned by the Len function, but what does this mean? So, if the Len function returns a value of four, the variable x will iterate from zero to three, taking the values zero, one, two, and three, and as you can see, it will iterate four times, as the Len function stated, if it returns a value of four.

The for block was then coded, which is a print, but in this case, "The sport" was printed, then it was concatenated with the string that returned the function STR(x+1), but why x+1? Because the first position of the sport will be zero as x goes from zero to the number that provides us the function range, we added one, and it will appear on the screen that the first sport is in position one. Following that, it is concatenated with "is" and with sport[x], in this case, as if it were a list, with the item of the position x of

the list, and these locations range from zero to the value n-1 of range.
Finally, the word "End" appeared on the screen, indicating that the program had completed and the for cycle had completed appropriately.

It's important to remember that in order for the variable x to change, it must iterate through a list, and as previously stated, the function range returns a list of m numbers, so if we say a = range (10), we can get a value of [0, 1, 2, 3, 4, 5, 6, 7, 8, 9], implying that the variable x will change from zero to nine.

b. Use Tuples in a "for" loop; tuples are sequence objects, and tuples are an immutable list data type, which means they can't be changed after they're created. This type of program is not difficult to create because programming in tuples and cycles is identical to programming in lists; the only difference is that the only thing to remember is to keep in mind.

Keep in mind the distinction between a list and a tuple.

Two examples will be presented in the same manner, the first with range and the second without this function.

1) Using Tuples and a range, loop for:

```python
foods=("pizza", "hot dog", "sushi")
x=0
for food in range(len(foods)):
    print("The x value is: "+str(x))
    print("The food value is: "+str(food))
    print("The foods item is: "+foods[food])
    x+=1
print("End")
```

The first thing we notice is that we construct the tuple foods, which contains several objects, like the strings "pizza," "hot dog," and "sushi," and as you should know, a tuple cannot be edited, changed, or anything like that after it is created.

Then a variable called x was declared, with the value zero.

The next step is to write the for loop, which, as you can see, will not iterate the variable x, but rather a food variable, which will iterate within the list that will return the range function, which should return a list of three elements, and why three elements? As you may know, the Len function returns the length of a list or tuple, and since the tuple foods contains three elements, the range function should produce a tuple with values ranging from zero to two.

Then, to see how the variable food iterates more clearly, the following instructions were programmed: first, the value of the variable x was printed in that instant, then, the value of food was printed in that instant, with the goal of verifying if they have the same value, and as you already know, the function str was used to concatenate an integer with a string. The next step is to print the associated food's item, which is why "The food item is:" is concatenated with foods [food], because we can select a specific value of the tuple foods, and in this case, it will be the one in the food position. Finally, it is stated that x will be adjusted to the following value.

To finish the code, the string "End" will be printed in the console to indicate that the program has completed and that it has completed correctly.

2) Loop with and without range for Tuples:

```python
messages=("Hello", "my", "name", "is", "Marco")
for message in messages:
    print(message)
print("End")
```

We can see that it is quite pleasant in this case because we send a message with the tuple, but how does this work? Well...

To begin, we build the tuple messages, which has the following items: "Hello," "my," "name," "is," and "Marco." As you can see, this is a five-item tuple, thus it has a length of five.

The next step is to design the for loop, which will run through the tuple messages; finally, the variable message will be written.

With it in this location, you may conclude that each message will be printed with a line break.

Finally, as in other examples, it will be printed in console "End" to indicate that it has completed the cycle and the program is complete.

c. Loop "for" with dictionary; the dictionary specifies a one-to-one relationship between keys and values, and dictionary type objects allow the Python interpreter to manipulate them using a set of operators.

Because all of these sorts of data are identical, this "for" loop with dictionary works similarly to the loops described above. However, they are different sorts of data and are processed differently, thus even if they are handled similarly, it is important to remember that they are different types of data.

Example:

```python
clothes={"shirt":"red", "shoes":"black","pant":"blue"}
for key in clothes:
    print(key)
clothe=input("Choose one of them: ")
if(clothe in clothes):
    print("Your clothe is "+clothe+" of color "+clothes[clothe])
else:
    print("Error")
```

With the variable we generated called clothing, which is a dictionary, we can see how to interact with dictionaries in this example. This includes the elements "shirt," which has a value connected with "red," "shoes," which has a value linked with "black," and "pant," which has a value associated with "blue."

The for cycle was then built, which tells us that the key variable would iterate through all of the values in the garments dictionary. And if you run this code in your favorite text editor, you'll notice that the key variable only has the values "shirt," "shoes," and "pant" associated with it. This is because the cycle inside the for prints the key-value inside the dictionary.

After that, we make the clothe variable, which is a variable that will receive an input from the user. When the user's value is received, an if is made, and if the variable clothe is inside clothes, as shown in the if's condition, it will be entered there, and it will be printed that "Your clothe is" + the user's option + "of color "+ clothes [clothe]; but what are clothes [clothe]? It's the value associated with the user's chosen clothe; for example, if the user selects "pant," clothes [clothe] will return the value "blue."

Finally, the otherwise condition says that if no clothe is found inside clothing, "Error" will be printed, which is very handy since if no value is found inside a database, an error will be thrown, regardless of whether the required value is found or not.

2. The "While" loop allows us to run cycles or periodic sequences that allow us to repeat a process several times. As long as the while condition is valid, and by true, we mean "True," this cycle will allow us to run a block indefinitely. This loop will be in charge of evaluating the condition, and if it is correct, the loop will be executed. At the end, the condition will be checked again, and if it is still true "True," the program will be executed again; if it is not true "False," the program will be executed once more.

There are various sorts of "while" loops, including the counting "while," the infinite while, and others, all of which are beneficial in specific situations.

It has a very simple syntax, which is as follows:
While (circumstance):
Within the cycle, there is a block of instructions.

Let's create a basic example in which the cycle prints a number as many times as the user desires.

Example:

```python
cycles=input("Put the number of cycles here: ")
count=0
while(count<int(cycles)):
    count+=1
    print("Cycle number "+str(count))
print("End")
```

We can see several things in this example. First, we create a variable cycles, which is an entry that will allow us, as users, to enter the number of cycles we want to do in this program. Of course, you must remember that this type of entry is a string, so you must transform it to perform mathematical operations.

Then another variable, count, will be created, with a vital function: it will be the cycle counter of our program, with which we will define that the same one will begin in zero, to begin the count.

The second step is to start the while cycle, as seen in the syntax above. First, we declare that we are going to make a while, and then we have the condition between the parentheses.

a. Counting loop; there is a counter in this cycle, and this counter will increase as the cycles are completed; this procedure will be done as many times as necessary until the expected number is attained. With the example we'll see next, we'll have a better understanding of this loop.

Despite the fact that we have previously seen an example of a while controlled by counting, that was the last one, it is never too much to take another example, this time using the counting method to make the counter go from higher to lower, as we will see below.

```python
1    cycles=input("Put the number of cycles here: ")
2    a=int(cycles)
3    while(0<a):
4        a-=1
5        print("Cycles to end "+str(a))
6    print("End")
```

In this case, we do a 180-degree turn because the counter does not have to reach its maximum value, but rather begins there and gradually decreases.

The first step is to establish a variable named cycles, which is linked to an input field that the user will fill in with the number of cycles he wishes to perform. The next step is to construct a variable a, which requires the function int () since it converts the variable cycles to an integer. As you may know, the variable cycles is a string because the entries are preserved that way, and arithmetic operations cannot be performed on strings.

The while loop is declared in the following line, and as can be seen, the condition is that zero must be strictly lower than a, therefore when an equals zero, the cycle will be exited and the other instruction will be passed.

The variable a must then be decreased within the cycle's block of instructions, which is accomplished by using the instruction a-=1, which is similar to saying that a = a -1, and can be easily observed as the variable an is reduced by one unit.

The next command is to output the message "Cycles to End" on the screen, followed by the number of missing cycles to exit the cycle.

Finally, the "End" string is displayed on the screen to indicate that the program is complete and that the while loop has been properly exited.

This type of cycle by counts is very useful; we'll start with the utility of those cycles in which the counter must grow; the first utility that comes to mind is to create a programmed chronometer that, when it reaches the maximum value, will exit the cycle and display on the screen that the required time has been met; now, there are other options. Now, while cycles per count are decreasing in this scenario, they may be used to create a countdown to sound an alarm or anything similar.

b. Infinite "while" loop: This sort of while is highly useful when an accumulation of instructions is performed an unknown number of times. In this situation, the programmer will make the condition a while (True), and as you can see, the True Boolean permits the while to work indefinitely.

Let's code two examples, one where we use an infinite while, the strict way, and one where we don't use the True condition to compel the block to be repeated forever, despite the fact that the programmer doesn't know the amount of cycles that will be done.

Examples:

1) In the case of the true situation:

```python
import time
x=1
while(True):
    print(x)
    x+=1
    time.sleep(1)
```

The first thing we notice is that the time module import is different, but those are issues we'll look into later; for now, it's not a big deal.

What actually interests us now is the declaration of the variable x as one, because it will act as a form of counter, gradually increasing.

The next step is to declare or create the while, and as you can see, the condition inside the while is True, so it will always be fulfilled, indicating that the cycle will be repeated at all times, unless some words are declared, as we shall see later.

The variable x will be printed on the screen inside the while block, and this is when it makes sense to utilize x as a counter since it will allow us to see in the console the exact second that has passed since the program began. The value of x is then increased since, as previously stated, it contains a counter function that grows one by one.

Finally, we utilize the library time, which causes a second delay. As a result, our software functions as a chronometer, displaying the second in which we are after running the code on the screen and updating it every second.

In the while loop, the following sentences are used:

1. Break Sentence: The term "break" is used to stop or abandon cycles that have not yet completed, implying that the evaluated expression of while remains in the true place. Let's look at an example to help you assess and comprehend this language.

```python
while True:
    x=input("Put one to break of the while cycle: ")
    if(x=="1"):
        break
    print("You dont put the one, please try again")
print("End")
```

We can understand how to construct unlimited while cycles in this example because, as you can see in the first line, the condition inside the while is always true, therefore we are in front of an infinite cycle.

Later, we declare the variable x, which is associated to the input function, which will wait for the user to enter any value, namely, a one, to exit the cycle; if the user enters anything other than the stated value, the cycle will be repeated.

As you can see in line three, you have an if statement that checks if x equals the string "1." Why is it being compared to a string? Because, as we already know, x is a string at the time this variable is declared because it is tied to the input function. If the condition is true, we'll utilize the "break" statement, which tells us to get out of the infinite loop.

If the condition is false, the following string will be written on the screen: "You don't put the one, please try again."

Finally, when the cycle is finished, the standard "End" will be printed to signal that the cycle was completed appropriately and the program was completed.

What can we learn from our break as an example? or what advantage can we derive from it? The first thing to understand is that the sentence break is particularly beneficial for breaking out of cycles; it does not have to be an absolutely infinite cycle because it may be employed in a cycle that is run by counting or another way. Another important feature is that this sort of sentence not only operates for a short period of time but can also be utilized in cycles, making it a valuable programming tool.

In what circumstances, though, should this form of statement be used? The first example that comes to mind is the handling of some exceptions that may arise within the cycles; if something unexpected happens, it exits the loop and either reports the error or does what you want it to do. Another example may be an access system, where a specific key has been requested, and if the proper key is not entered, the user will not be able to proceed to the next section of the application.

2. Sentence Continue: This sentence is particularly useful in programming because it allows us to omit what comes after the sentence in the cycle. That is, if some preceding

requirements are met, such as if we reach a continue sentence after numerous "if" or else, or other stages, we will skip the rest of the cycle's instructions and repeat the process. To summarize, if an instruction is repeated inside a loop, the interpreter is forced to return to the beginning of the loop, ignoring all of the instructions and interactions inside.

The following example shows a while cycle that ignores numbers that are multiples of five; if these values are multiples, they will not be written on screen, and the next iteration will be performed automatically.

```python
while.py
1    cycles=input("Please put the numer of cycles: ")
2    count=1
3    while(count-1<int(cycles)):
4        a=count
5        count+=1
6        if(a%5 == 0):
7            print("Error, continue")
8            continue
9        else:
10           print("Not is multiple of 5")
11       print(a)
12   print("End")
13
```

To begin, the variable cycles is created, which is an input that asks the user to enter the number of cycles he wants to do, and you have that cycles is a string, as you may know.

Then it generates the integer type variable count, which will have the role of a counter, allowing us to know where we are in the cycle and reach the maximum level that the user desires.

Now we'll make the while loop, which says that count-1 must be less than cycles, and why count -1? Because if the condition was lower or equal to cycles, the code would be less efficient, only a strict lower is used, and because the counter starts at one, it is required to subtract a unit and ensure that the number of matching cycles is met.

The variable an is defined in the next line, with the same count value, because we need to know the current value of the cycle, and, as you can see, the counter is increased by one unit, thanks to the instruction count += 1 in line 5.

After that, one enters the conditional block, where the condition is a percent 5 ==0 in this case, but what does this mean? To enter the if, the rest, which gives the division between a and five, must be strictly equal to zero. If the condition is true, the instructions in the if block will be carried out, which are as follows: the first step is to print an error message on the screen, after which the continue sentence will be utilized. If this condition is false, the instruction containing the else block, which notifies that the cycle is a multiple of five, will be passed.

The cycle number is presented on the screen at the end of the conditionals so we know where we are in the program.

Finally, a screen print is placed to demonstrate that the program has been completed and that the cycle has been properly exited.

What can we take away from this program now? The first is the use of the continue, because its function is to go directly to the next while cycle, omitting the other lines of the block. In this case, it is the same, because when we arrive at the continue, we pass to the other cycle, but if this sentence is not found, the value of a will be printed, as you can see.

3. Pass Sentence: It is a null expression, which means it does nothing, but it allows us to create a loop without placing code in its body so that we can add it later and use it as a temporary filler, which we mean to add some type of delay to the program; or it is a way to make a nop if you manage your programming with assembler or processors. It is a sentence that will not affect the behavior of the code in any way, and it should be noted that it can be used anywhere in the code without any problems, which means that the sentence can be used in a common function without any problems, but this is not worth mentioning yet because we have not seen functions, but it is not excessive to know that the pass can be implemented with functions. To establish a distinction, we may argue that continues will take care of finishing the current interaction but will continue with the next iteration of that loop, returning to the beginning, whereas pass would do nothing but continue with the following instructions without returning to the beginning. Let's have a look at an example of what it is.

```python
cycles=input("Please put the numer of cycles: ")
count=1
while(count-1<int(cycles)):
    a=count
    count+=1
    if(a%5 == 0):
        print("Error, continue")
        pass
    else:
        print("Not is multiple of 5")
    print(a)
print("End")
```

We can see how we define the variable cycles in the previous example, which will wait for the user to select how many cycles to utilize, and the input will be of the string type.

The count counter will then be established, which will begin at one for convenience but has the function of determining the cycle's current location.

The while cycle is created next, with the requirement that count-1 must be strictly less than int (cycles). It's worth noting that the int () function is used since the cycles variable is of string type, and comparisons between strings and integers are impossible due to the differing types of data. The rationale for the count- 1 is stated in the last example, so we won't go over it again. However, keep in mind that we're doing comparisons from zero, which is why the comparison is strictly lower and not lower or equal because we'd have to restart the cycle.

The following instructions define the variable a, which will be assigned the value of count, so that we can make operations on it without losing it; then the value of count will be increased by one unit, since if we don't, we'll be doing the same thing indefinitely.

The conditional phase is in charge of verifying if it is a multiple of five, and we do this by using the " percent " operator, which returns the rest of the division we place, so that if we place, for example, 10% 3, it will return the value of 1, which is the rest; similarly, when we put the following instruction a percent 5, we are asking for the rest between these values, and to know if a number is a multiple of five; in an analogous way, it is done here

Now, if the if condition is met, we will proceed to make a cumulus of instructions, the same as before, to print on screen that an error has been produced and that it will continue, then, the following instruction is the sentence pass, which will do nothing, is equivalent to causing a small delay in the program, depending on the frequency of the clock of our machine's processor. If the condition is false, however, it will be inserted into the else block, which will just print that the cycle number is not a multiple of five.

Now, whether the condition is true or false, the number of the cycle in which we are will be written on screen by the command print (a), because a represents the current position, at the time the conditional block was completed.

Finally, when the while loop is exited, the "End" string is written on the screen, indicating that the loop has been appropriately exited and the program is complete.

Now, if you're looking for a utility to the previous sentence, you won't find many right now if you haven't seen the functions, because it's just a delay right now, but it's not a delay that the user can notice because the computer clock frequency is in GHz, so it's so fast that it's not noticeable, but if you see the functions, there will be times when a complex program is being developed, and there are parts that haven't.

Chapter 5: Functions

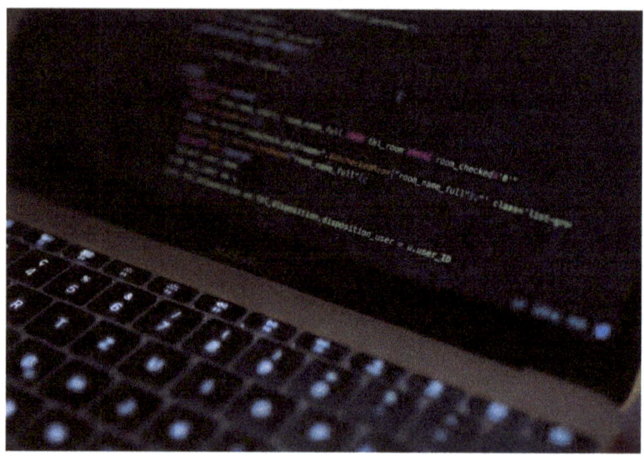

A function is essentially a chunk or block of reusable code that accomplishes a certain goal. It is a code block with a name that accepts inputs as input, as well as a sequence of words that executes a desired operation, returns a result, and performs a task. This block may be called whenever we need it, which is a significant benefit. Python is a language that allows us to create these functions with a lot of freedom.

The use of these functions is a fundamental component of the structured programming paradigm, and thus offers various advantages:

* Because it permits reusing the same function in different programs, it eliminates the need to duplicate the code several times while performing the functions. It helps us to break down a big program into smaller modules, making programming easier and debugging

easier; as the expression goes, "divide and conquer." As a result, it is a widely utilized approach.

The Python programming language has what are known as functions, which allow us to create functions specified by the user and use them later in his own application.

The following are the functions:

Function	Use	Example	Result
Print ()	This function allows the program to	Print ("Hello")	"Hello"

	print in screen the desired argument		
Len ()	This function allows you to determine the length of the characters that a string contains	Len ("Hello world")	11
Join()	This function allows you to convert a string to another by using "-"	List=['Python', 'is'] '- '. Join (List)	'Python-is'
Split()	This function will let you convert a string into a list	A=("This will be a list") List2= a.split()	A=['This', 'will', 'be', 'a', 'list']
Replace()	This function, as it names indicates, will let you replace a string for another	Text= "The house is green" Print (Text) Text= Text.replace("green", "yellow") Print(Text)	"The house is green" "The house is yellow"
Upper() and lower()	This function allows us to	Text= "The house is green"	"THE HOUSE IS

		convert into upper or lower case all the letters in a string	Text.upper() Print (Text) Text.lower() Print(Text)	GREEN" "the house is green"
Ord()	This function will let you use ASCII data type	Print (ord('A'))	65
Tuple()	This function will convert a string into a tuple	Words= tuple ("I am old") Print(Words)	('I', 'a', 'm', 'o', 'l', 'd')
Type()	This function will return the type of data of an element	X=5 Print(type(X))	<class 'int'>
List ()	This function will let you create lists from an element	Word= list('Hello') Print (Word)	['H', 'e', 'l', 'l', 'o']
Round ()	This function will round the decimal part of a number to its nearest integer	Print (round(15,746))	16
Str()	This function will convert a	X=5 A=str(X)	"5"

		numerical value into a string	Print (A)	
Range()	This function will create a list of n elements. It is mainly used in the for cycle	X=range(3) Print(X)	[0, 1, 2]
Float ()	This function will allow us to convert any value to a decimal type of value	A=float("5.55") Print(A)	5.55
Max() & Min()	These functions will determinate the higher and the lower values in a set of numbers	X= [2, 6, 3, 8, 0] Print (max(X)) Print(min(X))	8 0
Sum()	This function will add the numbers of a set of numbers	X=[3, 1, 6] Print(sum(X))	10
Int()	This function will convert any value into an integer	A=("35") Print (int(A))	35

What guidelines must I follow in order to define a function?

- The function's input parameters must be defined within the function's parenthesis.
- When writing the code, we must correctly and thoroughly identify the indentation (4 characters of space).
- After we put the colon, the function's code will always begin. ": It should be emphasized that a function will not be run until it is invoked, and that a function must be called by its name in order to be invoked. Consider the following scenario:

```python
a=[1, 2, 3, 4, 5]
b=[1, 0, 1, 0, 1]
num="5 6 7 8 9"
c=num.split()
print(c)
e=[]
for x in c:
    d=int(x)
    e.append(d)
c=e
d=[]
for x in range(len(a)):
    e=a[x]+b[x]+c[x]
    d.append(e)
e=min(d)
f=max(d)
g=sum(d)
print(a)
print(b)
print(c)
print(d)
print(e)
print(f)
print(g)
```

As we can see in this example, we generated variables a and b, which are lists of integer values, particularly five items, an is a list of numbers ranging from one to five, and b is an iteration of one and zero values.

The second step is to create the variable num, which is a string with the value "5 6 7 8 9," and as we previously saw, the function split () creates an arrangement of strings, each item being a word separated by white space. We use this function in the code, specifically in line four, to convert the variable c into a list of strings with the value ["5", "6", "7", "8", "9"], but it is not possible to perform mathematical operations with it.

To accomplish our goal, we first declare the variable e as an empty list, and then we use a for loop in which the variable x iterates through the array c, which has its items as strings, and thus within a variable d, the integer returned by applying the function int () to the element of the list c at that time. Then, within the list e, the value of d is added until the number of iterations has reached its maximum. The next step is to save the list that was previously saved in e in c, so that the variables are in a more logical sequence.

In order to store data in the variable d, it was given the value of an empty list. Then, with the help of a for, which will iterate as many times as the number of items in the list a, as we will have to move through all of its items, since what we want to do is create another list that contains the sum of a, b, and c, it is said that e will be equal to the sum of the item in position x, of lists a, b, and c, so inside the same buffer, it is said that e will be The append function will be used to append the value received to the d list after the three items have been added.

What is the best way to make your own function?

To be able to build our own function, we must use the "def." sentence to name it, however this time it will not be the name of a preset function; instead, it will be a name that we have generated.

What is the best way to invoke a function?

We just need to declare a function when we begin writing our code to be able to invoke it. This is critical because a function that has not been constructed in advance cannot be called. Example:

Parameters

A parameter is a type of value that is passed into a function when it is called. A function can take one or more parameters. In order for these parameters to be invoked, they must be separated by a comma "." Example:

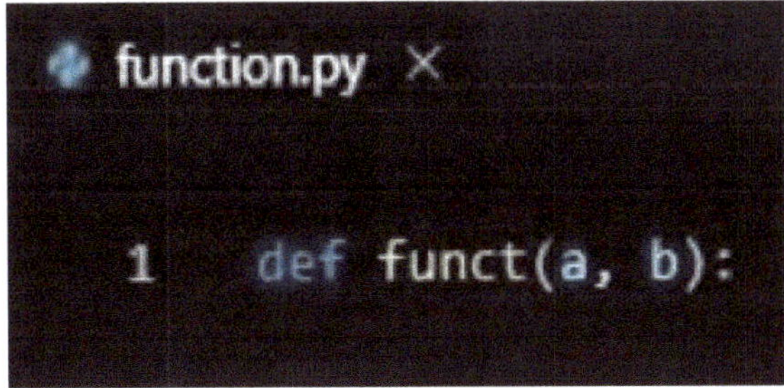

As you can see in this short example, it's only to explain how the first component of a function should be defined, which is why it's so easy.

The def., which defines that a function will be formed or, to put it another way, signals that a function is being defined, is a statement that must never be omitted when declaring a function.

Then there's a word, in this case funct, which was used to give our function a name, and then there's a parenthesis with two letters, a and b, which denotes the parameters that our function would receive in order to function.

What are the best ways to define parameters and arguments?

The values that the function receives when it is defined are referred to as arguments. These values are referred to as arguments and are separated into types when the function is invoked.

Several forms of arguments exist:

Arguments by name:

When calling a function, the value of each parameter must be specified in the arguments, commencing with the name of the parameter.

```python
1    def funct(a, b):
2        return a+b
3
4    c=funct(b=5, a=3)
5    print(c)
6
```

As can be seen, we're still using the funct function, with the same parameters a and b. We can also see how the definition is same, with the exception of line two, which shows that the sum of a and b will return. The return sentence will be discussed later, but it is not overly complicated; its name tells us exactly what it does, which is to return a value.

The variable c is then created in the following lines, and it will be equal to the value returned by the function we just built, as well as the sum of its parameters a and b, as previously stated. As you can see, when you call the function in line four, you first write the function's name, in this case funct, and then the arguments that will be passed are previously specified with the name, as you can see, the argument with a value of five is specified as parameter b of the funct function, and similarly with parameter a.

Finally, the value of c is displayed on the screen, allowing you to confirm that the result is correct.

Argument by position:
When we provide an argument to a function, the defined parameters are sent to them in the order they were defined.

```python
def hello(name, color):
    print("Hello "+name+ " your favorite color is "+color)


a=input("What is your name? ")
b=input("What is your favorite color? ")
hello(a,b)
```

Another function, named hello, will be built in this example, with the parameters name and color. This function will be used to create a screen message in which the user will be greeted by his name and told what color he prefers.

To call this function, first declare two variables. The first is variable a, which is responsible for storing the value of the string related to the user's name, and the second is variable b, which is responsible for storing the string related to the user's favorite color. Both variables are related to the input function, which means they will be waiting for the user to enter the value he desires.

Finally, the greeting function is called with its name, but the parameters were supplied by order rather than by name, so you must pay close attention to the exact order, since if you make a mistake, the program can easily collapse or fail to perform the task.

As you can see, there are several methods for passing arguments; you can use whichever method you prefer; if you find it easier or faster to pass arguments by position, do so, but keep in mind that you must ensure that the argument is in the correct parameter position; if you prefer to pass arguments by name, do so, but keep in mind that you must ensure that the parameter names are written correctly.

Call without arguments

If some defined parameters are not given correctly when calling a function, an error will be generated.

```
function.py  ×

1    def hello():
2        print("Hello")
3
4    hello()
```

The hello function is constructed in this example, which will not take any parameters and will merely print the message "Hello" on the screen.

Then, in order to call it, only the function's name will be written in parenthesis, as follows: name ().

Return Statement

Most Python functions have a return value, which can be explicit or implicit, as we've seen earlier.

Return is a reserved word whose purpose is to complete the execution of a function and then return the value returned as a result. If you want to see an example of this, look at the one in arguments by position, where you can see that the function has a return sentence that returns the value of the sum of a plus b; and also, as you can see in this example, that value is saved in the variable c, which is then printed.

Lambda Function

Lambda functions are a subset of Python's predefined functions. So, what exactly do we mean? Because it has a fairly exclusive syntax, this sort of function is known for being "exclusive" because it allows us to easily generate "anonymous" functions.

Lambda functions can execute an expression and return its result; they can also have optional parameters in their structure, but they come with their own set of constraints.

The lambda function's syntax is described below.

The lambda function in Python has a relatively basic syntax, requiring simply the use of the reserved word lambda, followed by the action's arguments, and finally the double point ":" to separate them.

```
function.py ×

1    sum= lambda x,y: x+y
2    a=sum(3,10)
3    print(a)
```

In this example, we learn how to utilize the lambda function, and in this case, the sentence lambda, to create a function that sums two numbers, x and y. As a result, we notice that the parameters we have are x and y; as a result, return the sum of both inside the function's block.

Finally, to invoke the function, we assigned the value that returns sum to the variable a, and then, to ensure that the result is certain, we printed the value that stores the variable a on the screen, and if you execute this program, you will notice that it returns 13.

The lambda function is frequently used when you need to call a function for a brief period of time (it doesn't require a name) and is frequently combined with the integrated functions filter () and map () ().

Filter Function ()

As its name implies, the filter () function is in charge of filtering. What exactly does that imply? This function accepts a list or an iterator as an argument and returns an iterable with the entries already filtered (this will return a true if the condition is met).

```
function.py

1    def pair(n):
2        if(n>0 and n%2==0):
3            return True
4        else:
5            return False
6
7    numbers=[]
8    for x in range(25):
9        numbers.append(x)
10
11   pairs=filter(pair, numbers)
12
13   for x in pairs:
14       print("The number "+str(x)+" is pair")
15
```

For this example, the first thing we need is a conditional function to know what we're going to filter; in our case, we'll create the pair function, which will have the integer n as a parameter; next, we'll enter a conditional block, where the condition is that n must be greater than zero, because zero is an odd number; and the other condition is that the remainder of the division between n and two has to be even; finally, we'll enter a conditional block

The next step is to populate the variable numbers, which will be an empty list, with our arrangement of numbers that we will filter. The range function, which gives us the for loop's bounds, is then used to enter a for loop, in which a variable x will fluctuate from zero to 24, as seen in line 8. The next step is to fill in our list using the append function in the numbers variable, which, as you may recall, is an empty list that, once filled in, becomes a list with integer values as items.

We can already filter the list by creating a list called pairs, which will use the filter function and return the values of the arrangement that the function returns to us as True, as in example 2, because this one is greater than zero and the module of the division of the same one, between two, is zero, it meets the requirements.

The next step is to print all of the obtained pairings on the screen, which we achieve with the help of another cycle for, in which a variable x iterates over the entire list and prints us that all of the numbers are even.

Function Map ()

The map () function is responsible for executing each member of a list or tuple in order to return a sequence of elements as the outcome of the operation.

```python
def sum(a, b):
    return a + b


list1=[1, 0, 1, 0, 1]
list2=[0, 2, 0, 2, 0]
c=map(sum, list1, list2)
print(list(c))


string1=["Hello, ", "are "]
string2=["how ","you"]
c=map(sum, string1, string2)
print(list(c))
```

In the initial lines of this example, we can see the creation of a function named sum, which takes two parameters, a and b, which do not have to be integers but can be strings or any other sort of data. Whether it's a concatenation or a sum, it'll return a+b.

Later, we generated two lists, "List1" and "List2," which are identical in that they each contain an iteration of numbers between one and zero, in the case of List1, and iterations between the numbers two and zero in the case of List2.

Then we declare a variable c, which will use the map function and receive as arguments the functions sum, list1, and list2. What this will do is build a list in a certain memory address, with the total of list1 and list2 as elements. It is critical to use the list() sentence to print what is in c, since we must notify the computer that we want to see the list that is in that memory address if we want to see the desired data.

Later, two variables were defined: string1 and string2, the latter of which will hold a message. Following the declarations, the map variable is used, using the arguments sum, string1 and string2. In this case, we're concatenating the strings that make up each list item. Finally, we'll print the value of the list in address c on the screen.

What are the distinctions between lambda functions and functions specified using the "def." sentence?

We already know that the "def." statement may be used to build functions built with the lambda function. What exactly does this imply? This simply indicates that using either of these two statements to create a function is a correct activity. This is because both procedures yield the same result, albeit with fewer possibilities.

We may think of this as two paths that both lead to the same place; the difference is that one is longer and heavier, while the other is much simpler, which is exactly what the lambda function is for: to make it easier to use functions in our code.

In contrast to the def. statement, which typically consumes several times more than one line of code, when we build a lambda type function, it will only focus on utilizing a single line of code, minimizing the number of lines that can be utilized in a code.

Unlike the def. statement, which must be defined at the beginning of the program so that it can be interpreted, the lambda keyword creates an object or function that does not require a name to be defined.

Although the code is shorter when utilizing the lambda function, the def. statement is often more clear for those who are new to programming or who have some programming knowledge but not much expertise.

It is critical to assign a variable to the lambda function when using it, because if this is not done, the lambda function will only act in the line in which it is declared.

Chapter 6:
Object-Oriented
Programming (OOP).

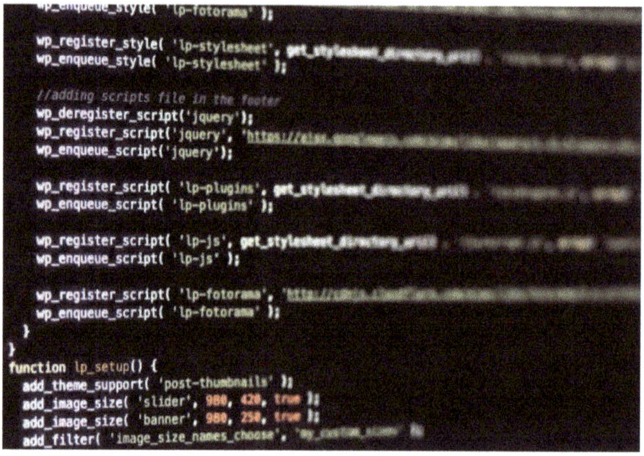

We can already create the program based on functions at this level, allowing us to utilize statements to change the data. Procedure-oriented programming and object-oriented programming are two forms of programming that employ types defined by the programmer to arrange both codes and data in this programming language.

What is OOP and what are the benefits of using it?

It is a type of programming utilized by modern languages that involves translating the behavior of real-world objects to programming code. It's a method of arranging your program by enclosing it in an object, which combines data and functionality. Python, C++, Java, Visual, and other programming languages use the object-oriented paradigm.

We can list the following benefits: - We can divide programs into chunks, parts, modules, or classes, which is known as modularization in programming.

- Unlike procedure-oriented programming, it is code that can be reused, therefore if we construct an application using this object-oriented program and later wish to create another comparable application, we can reuse this code. Now, in order to reuse code from one application in another, we must first learn and comprehend the idea of "inheritance."
- If a line of code fails, the program will continue to run; however, the line of code that caused the mistake is unlikely to complete the intended goal, but the rest of the program will.

Encapsulation is a term used to describe the act of enclosing something

Object-oriented programming entails the use of programming concepts such as:

a. Abstraction: Abstraction refers to a design and interpretation process that focuses on detecting the key properties of an object while filtering out and ignoring the details that aren't significant.

Abstraction is concerned with establishing the qualities of an object that set it apart from others. It describes what it should be implemented in after focusing on what it is rather than what it accomplishes.

For instance, we'll use abstraction to create flowers.
Object: Flowers Characteristics
- Colors
- Leaves
 - Nectar

- Roots

Functionalities:
- Seeds and fruits production
- Cross-pollination
- Propagation

b. Inheritance: certain objects inherit properties and methods from other objects, as well as adding new ones. We call this inheritance, a class that inherits from another, similar to how one of the children in a family group inherits the skin color of one of the parents, and he would be inheriting or having their own features or properties, but also one in common with one of their parents.

What exactly does this imply? To put it another way, when we build a new class, we can use the same data as the base class. This new class will include more detailed data than the old class, which has a broader view.

When a class in Python doesn't inherit from another, it must inherit from an object, which is the fundamental Python class that defines an object.

It is possible to access an object's method and properties once it has been formed, or once a class instance has been generated, and Python employs a very simple syntax for this: the object's name, followed by the point, and the property or method you want to access.

Multiple inheritances are also supported in Python, albeit only to a limited extent.

Inheritance types include:

- Basic Inheritance: When a class inherits only one base class, this is known as basic inheritance.

- Multiple inheritance: When a class inherits from two or more base classes, this is known as multiple inheritance.

- Polymorphism: This term refers to the various behaviors that are linked to things that are diverse but have the same name. When you call an object by its name (which may contain many objects), its behavior is determined by the object you are currently using.

Polymorphisms are classified as follows:

- Parametric polymorphism: Parametric polymorphism is a sort of polymorphism that allows functions and classes to be defined in a generic manner, allowing data to be modified without regard to type.

- Polymorphism of subtypes: Polymorphism of subtypes is when the subtypes of a type (class) allow for the substitution of an own implementation for the behavior of the original type's functions.

- Ad Hoc Polymorphism: Ad Hoc polymorphism refers to functions that behave differently depending on the type of arguments they receive.

What language or vocabulary will we use in OOP?

To help you grasp this code, we'll go over the most regularly used vocabulary:

```python
class house():
    color="red"
    dors=6
    kitchen=True
    bathroom=3
    levels=2

house1=house()
print("We create a house")
```

- Class: Classes are models on which objects are formed, that is, models that include the common properties of a group of things. We will use analogies to better comprehend this phrase. For example, if we have a car, the class would be the chassis and wheels, because this is a common property across the group of things that are cars. If we want to make a Python program that makes vehicles, we must first establish a class that identifies the common qualities of the cars we want to make, as well as the building of a chassis and four wheels.

To demonstrate another abstraction, let's utilize a class example, except this time the class will be a house.

The first step, as shown in the example, is to declare that home is a class by using the reserved term class. It has some characteristics, such as being red, having six doors, having a kitchen, having three bathrooms, and having two stores.

The next step is to establish a variable and convert it to a class. For this, any name can be used, and then the class name and parenthesis are added. As you can see in the example, house1 is an object with a house class and all of the previously mentioned characteristics.

Finally, to see if the class was properly constructed, a print is made in the console to check the program's appropriate operation.

- Exemplar of class, which is synonymous with instance of class and object belonging to a class, implying that exemplar, instance, and object of class are interchangeable terms; an instance would be an object or exemplar belonging to a class. Following the example of the automobile, we've already discussed how the class defines the characteristics that are common to it, as well as the objects that we'll use, and how the class is formed in our example by the chassis and wheels, but the objects that belong to that class could be different models of automobiles that share a common characteristic.

- Modularization; when we create a complex application applied to objects such as Python, for example, the most common is that this application is composed of several classes, not a single class, which can also occur, but the most common is that if the application is complex, it will be composed of several classes. The concept of modularization derives from the fact that an application can be composed of several classes, for example, if we imagine an old sound symphony. These modules have the advantage of being self-contained; for example, if the radio was broken, we could use the cassette module; similarly, if you have a Python program divided into modules and one of the classes fails for any reason, the program will most likely continue to run; however, the class in which you have problems will not be able to carry out its task, as with the analogy of the sound eq.

- Encapsulation; the internal functioning of a complete class of our object-oriented program is encapsulated, which means that the other classes do not handle any information about each other; returning to the sound equipment analogy, the internal functioning of the equalizer corresponds only to the equalizer, meaning the functioning of the cassette module; nothing knows or understands the equalizer module. All of the classes are connected in some way so that they function as equipment,   but each class is also encapsulated so that the internal workings of that class are not visible from the outside. With something called access methods, the various sections of a program are linked together to form a team. We can connect one class to another and have them work as a unit or a team by creating access methods, however these access methods will only have access to certain features of each of the classes. You can move from one class to another to connect them, but certain characteristics of each class are contained and therefore not accessible.

In Python, how can we create classes, objects, and access an object's properties and characteristics?

We utilize what is known as nomenclature of the point, which is often used in object-oriented programming, to access the features and characteristics of an object. To clarify what it is, we will use an example.

Assume we've given our object a name, such as myCar; all objects, instances, or exemplars must have a name. To access the car's properties in our application, we'll use the point nomenclature:
E.g. Syntax: The object's name. New Value = Property

MyCar.
Color="red"

In Python, this is the syntax to employ if we wish to access an object's property; we utilize the point's nomenclature. The point nomenclature is also used to access the object's functionality from the code.

Syntax: Object name. Behavior, for example.
myCar.starts ()
myCar.stops ()

To help you understand better, the following example will show you how to access the characteristics of a class using the point nomenclature.

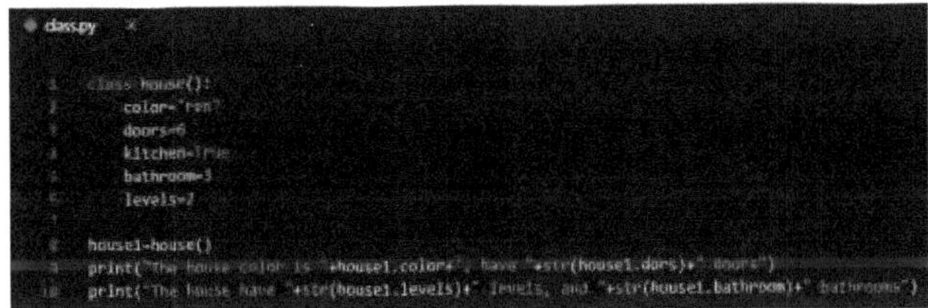

```python
class house():
    color="red"
    doors=6
    kitchen=True
    bathroom=3
    levels=2

house1=house()
print("The house color is "+house1.color+", have "+str(house1.dors)+" doors")
print("The house have "+str(house1.levels)+" levels, and "+str(house1.bathroom)+" bathrooms")
```

The first thing we see in this example is the construction of the house class, which has its own set of properties, such as the color, which is red in this case, the number of doors, which is six, and the number of floors, which is two.

Then we'll see how to make our house1 instance, which belongs to the house type. However, we do not only want to stay with the creation of the class; we also want to access the data that these have, so we will make a screen print of the attributes that the house has, as you can see, what we proceed to do is concatenate the string that we have written with the attribute we want, now, to access it, we must name the instance, and through the nomenclature of the point, the attribute we want to access.

Now we'll look at how to establish a class in code, with the class serving as the foundation for later creation of objects, examples, and instances that belong to that class.

```
class.py        ×

1     class obj():
2             <statement 1>
3             .
4             .
5             .
6             .
7             .
8             <statement n>
9
10    a=obj()
11
```

This is more than an example; it is an explanation of the syntax for declaring a class, because, despite being redundant, declaring them is a key part of object-oriented programming, because, as you may have guessed, it is the foundation. As a result, the first step is to create the class name object () statement: with this, we are establishing a class named name object. Then there is a cumulus of statements inside it that are responsible for assigning values to the attributes of the instances and working with the methods that will be detailed later.

There will be times when you will wonder, "But all the houses are red, or all the trees have three leaves?" And, clearly, the answer is no; for this, we will collaborate with the builders, who will allow us to give each instance its own identity. These are methods, but there's no need to go into detail because they're the ones that allow us to assign different values to each instance at the time of initialization; we'll look at them later.

Despite the fact that you should already know what an attribute is because we've already discussed it,

We've already worked with them in this chapter; now we'll go over them in detail.

Attribute: Within each object, we specify attributes as the values that variables have. What exactly do we mean when we say this? Consider the scenario of a classroom in a school; one of the characteristics that each classroom may have is the students' grade or age.

The term attribute can be applied to anything that comes after a point. For example, in the expression z.real, real is an attribute of the object z, which we earlier referred to as the point nomenclature.
Read-only or write-only properties are available. The assignment of characteristics is possible in this last situation. A module's attributes can be written as follows: These properties can be erased with the Del instruction if needed. Module. The answer = 42 consider the following: The attribute the answer of the object with module name will be removed with Del module.the answer.

```
  class.py        ×

1     class house():
2         color="red"
3         dors=6
4         kitchen=True
5         bathroom=3
6         levels=2
7
8     house1=house()
9     house1.color="green"
10    print(house1.color)
11
```

The first step in this example is to construct the class house (), and then to define each of its attributes, such as color, bathroom, and kitchen, among others.

The next step is to create the house1 instance, which is of the house type, as you might assume. However, if you want to paint the house, we'll access the attribute by using the instruction house1.color = "green," which changes the color from house1 to "green."
A screen print of the color attribute of the house1 instance is made using the dot nomenclature to ensure that the color has been altered correctly.

Methods:

We'll call methods to each function generated within each class now that we've seen that each object has various characteristics that have certain behavior. What are your thoughts on this? So, returning to the classroom as an example, it has two techniques or actions: studying and attending classes.

We use the term def. to construct a method, which we already know, but when we write it, there is a keyword that we must remember, which a parameter of the function is, and this word is self, and it is used to access the class's attributes. We can see that there is a distinction between method and function, with a method being a particular function that belongs to the class being constructed, whilst a function does not.

The reserved word def. the name of the function, and a default parameter called self are the characteristics of a method.

The method's first argument is frequently referred to as self. This is just a convention; the name self means nothing to Python in the sense that it doesn't matter whether you put it as the first or last parameter (because the order doesn't matter, but it has to be the word self), but if you don't follow it, your code may be less readable to other Python programmers.

If the notion of attributes is fully understood, we can see that working with methods is relatively straightforward; however, when working with them, we must remember that methods are used to add behavior to objects, allowing you to alter attributes when visiting a method or returning a value.

```python
class house():
    color="red"
    dors=6
    kitchen=True
    bathroom=3
    levels=2

    def open(self):
        print("The door is open")
house1=house()
house1.color="White"
print(house1.color)
house1.open()
```

We see how to create the class house in this example,
but it differs from the others because it has created a
different method, called open. As you can see, it uses the
sentence def., then the name of the method, then the
parameters, always, but always, the self as a parameter,
you can add others, but the self cannot be missed. After
then, it's treated like any other function; as you can see,
the method's job is to send a message indicating that the
door is open.

Later on, you'll see how to create the instance house1,
which is a subclass of house. One of the first things you'll
notice is that you can change the color of house1, which
is now white. Another important action is access to the
methods, which, as you can see, is also done using the
dot nomenclature.

Constructors:

Now that you have a basic understanding of classes, you should consider whether all instances of one class are the same, because if this were the case, everything would be very monotonous, and the OOP would not be as powerful as it is. As a result, constructors were created, which initialize the classes with the values that the programmer desires.

A constructor is a method that creates or assigns values to an instance's initial attributes, and to do so, we use the reserved word init (self, a, b, c,...), where a, b, c are the parameters that we want to initialize, and thus be able to assign values to the attributes, in order to achieve diversity in our init (self, a, b, c,...)

```python
class house():
    def __init__(self, color, dors, kitchen, bathroom, levels):
        self.color=color
        self.dors=dors
        self.kitchen=kitchen
        self.bathroom=bathroom
        self.levels=levels

    def open(self):
        print("The door is open")

    def paint(self, c):
        self.color=c
house1=house("blue", 5, True, 2, 1)
print(house1.color)
house1.paint("black")
print(house1.color)
house1.open()
```

We can observe how things change and become more enjoyable in this example. The first thing to notice is that a constructor was used, which has as parameters the self, color, doors, and kitchen, among others. We use the word self after the constructor's statement and place the corresponding value, as you can see between lines three and seven. For example, in the instruction on line 3, it says that the variable color of that specific instance will have the value that the argument had when the instance was initialized.

Then you can see how the open method was created; that method only shows on screen that the door has been opened; the other method that has been created, in this case, is paint, which is responsible for changing the color of that instance; this was done using the sentence self. Color to specify that the instance will change.

Following that, the house1 instance is constructed and passed to the constructor as an argument "blue", 5, True, 2, 1 so that he can initialize his attributes with those precise values and thus break the monotony.

After creating the instance, the color of the house is printed in screen, or more precisely, the color of the house1 instance, which should print the string "blue" at this time. It then uses the paint method to change the color of the instance to black, and to verify that the color has been changed correctly, the color of the house1 instance is printed in screen, and in this case, the string "black" should appear in console.

Finally, the open method is utilized to make the doors appear to be open on the screen.

Because we know how to use the builders, we can use the inheritance idea we learned earlier to ensure that a class associated to it inherits the behaviors and properties of its parent class.

```python
class house():
    def __init__(self, color, dors, kitchen, bathroom, levels):
        self.color=color
        self.dors=dors
        self.kitchen=kitchen
        self.bathroom=bathroom
        self.levels=levels

    def open(self):
        print("The door is open")

    def paint(self, c):
        self.color=c
class apartment(house):
    def __init__(self, color, dors, kitchen, bathroom, levels, stairs, elevator):
        house.__init__(self, color, dors, kitchen, bathroom, levels)
        self.stairs=stairs
        self.elevator=elevator
    def elevatoron(self):
        if(self.elevator==True):
            print("The elevator is in PB")
        else:
            print("You dont have elevator")
house1=house("blue", 5, True, 2, 1)
print(house1.color)
house1.paint("black")
print(house1.color)
house1.open()
apartment1=apartment("orange", 2, True, 2, 1, True, True)
apartment1.elevatoron()
apartment1.open()
```

We can see how inheritance works in this example, but since we've previously seen the first lines of code, we won't go over them in detail. All we do is build the house class, initialize the house constructor, and add some methods like paint and open.

The second class, which is apartments, is then defined. Why do we call her a daughter of the house class? We already know that an apartment is a house, but a home does not have to be an apartment; it might be a mansion or a townhouse, for example, so it is not necessarily true.

As can be seen, when defining the apartment class, we pass the parent class, in this example, house, as a parameter. Then we start the constructor, which should have the reserved word __init__, and pass in the parameters self and all that are missing, which includes both the parameters of the class house's entry as well as any additional parameters of the class apartment, such as stairs and elevators, since apartments can have or not have stairs. They, too, must be initialized. Later, as we can see, we will call the parent class's function of constructors, so that the same ones are initialized, using the dot nomenclature, and then it is when the other non-house attributes, such as stairs or elevator, are initialized. The elevator on() method was built within the apartment class, and when called, it will appear on screen that the elevator is on the ground floor, depending on whether the instance produced contains an apartment or not.

After creating all of the classes, we proceed to create the instances to ensure that the classes were created correctly. In a similar manner to how the object house1 was created, this one is created, with the same values as the previous example, the object's color is printed, the color is changed to black using the function paint(), and the door is finally opened. Then there's the apartment1, which has the orange hue as an argument, two doors, True on the kitchen, two baths, one level, stairs, and an elevator. The function elevator on () is invoked in the software to summon the elevator and get to the bottom floor, and to indicate the user that this is in PB. After that, the open method is used to open the apartment doors.

As we can see, object-oriented programming is extremely useful because it allows us to see programming problems as real-life problems and create solutions as if they were objects we encounter in everyday life. As a result, we strongly recommend programming this way because it reduces the number of lines used, makes the code reusable, and is easier to understand.

Chapter 7:
Modules

Modules are files with the extension.py (which we have been using until now), but they can also be files with the extension.pyc (which is a compiled Python file), or a file written entirely in C for people who use CPython. Modules have their own namespace and can contain variables, functions, classes, and even other modules, either as a sub module or a module within a module.

What value do the modules provide?

The modules are mostly used to organize and reuse code, which brings us to two key terms in OOP: modularization and reuse. One of the advantages of modules is that they allow us to reuse our code in other applications when we wish to develop a complicated application and need functionality that was previously programmed in another application. When we realize a complex program, we may do it in a single file with thousands of lines of code, or we can divide it into little pieces, in small files with a smaller number of lines of code, because it will always be easier for us to handle.

In Python, how do we make a module?

We can easily construct a module using the.py file extension, and we can then save it wherever we want, which is known as import.

Python's standard library has a vast number of modules; we may find this library by going to http://docs.python.org/modindex.html in the official Python manual.

The name of a module can be found in the value of the global variable _name_.

Sentence of Importance

A module can contain executable statements and function definitions; we can initialize the module using these statements. They are only run the first time a module is used in an import statement.

Modules have the ability to import other modules. All import declarations are usually placed at the beginning of the module (or script, for that matter). The names of the imported modules will be stored in the importing module's global namespace.

The syntax of the import sentence is as follows:
If the module is present in the search path when the interpreter discovers the import line, it will be imported.

A search path is nothing more than a list of directories that the interpreter searches for before importing a module.

Chapter 8:
File management

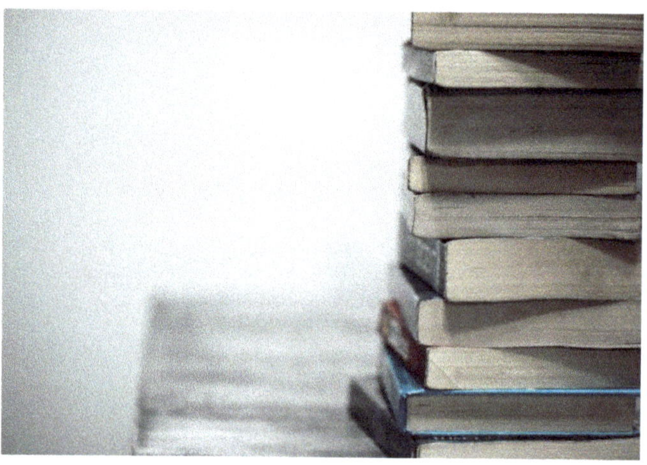

When it comes to file systems and directories, the Python programming language allows us to work on two levels. One of these is via the os module, which allows us to operate with the entire system of files and directories at the operating system level.

The second level enables us to work with files by altering their reading and writing at the application level, as well as treating each file as an object.

The files are manipulated in three steps in python, as well as any other language: first they are opened, then they are operated on or altered, and finally they are closed.

What exactly is a file?

A python file is a collection of bytes that form a structure. Within this structure, we find the header, which contains all of the file's data, such as the name, size, and type of file we're working with; the data is part of the body of the file, which contains the written content, which is handled by the editor; and finally, the end of the file, which informs the code that we've reached the end of the file. We can explain the structure of a file in this way.

The following is the order in which the files are organized:

- File headers: These are the data that will be contained in the file (name, size, type)

- File Data: This is the file's main body, and it will contain some content produced by the programmer.

- End of file: This sentence signifies that the file has reached its conclusion.

This is how our file will look:

**Header of file
(name, size, type)**

Body of file (data)

End of file

How can I gain access to a file?

There are two main methods for accessing a file: one is to treat it as a text file and go line by line, and the other is to treat it as a binary file and go byte by byte.

To assign a file type value to a variable, we'll need to use the open () function, which allows us to open a file.

Open () function

To open a file in Python, we must use the open () function, which takes as parameters the file name and the method by which the file will be opened. If the file opening mode is not specified, it will open as a read-only file by default.

It's important to remember that the file actions are limited since you can't read a file that was only opened for writing, and you can't write to a file that was only opened for reading.

The open () function has two parameters:
- The path to the file we want to open;
- It's the mode in which it can be accessed.

It has the following syntax:

```
1    function = open("file.txt", "w")
2    function.write()
3    function.close()
```

The following are the parameters:

File: This is an argument that specifies the name of the file we wish to open with the open () method; the path of our file will be specified by this argument.
The argument file is regarded a basic argument because it is the most important (enabling us to open the file), as opposed to the other arguments, which can be optional and have fixed values.

Mode: The access modes are the ones in charge of determining how the file will be opened (it could be for reading, writing, editing).

There are several modes of access available, including:

r	This is the default open mode. Opens the file for reading only
r+	This mode opens the file for its reading and writing
rb	This mode opens the file for reading only in a binary format
w	This mode opens the file for writing only. In case the file does not exist, this mode creates it
w+	This is similar to the w mode, but this allows the file to be read
wb	This mode is similar to the w mode, but this opens the file in a binary format
wb+	This mode is similar to the wb mode, but this allows the file to be read
a	This mode opens a file to be added. The file starts writing from the end
ab	This is similar to mode a, but opens the file in a binary format
a+	This mode is pretty much like the mode a, but allows us to read the file.

In conclusion, there are three letters, or three primary modes: r, w, and a. There are also two sub modes, + and b.

Text files and plain files are the two types of files in Python. To avoid any errors in our code, it's critical to declare the format the file will be opened in.

Read a document:
A file can be read in three ways:
1. read ([n])
2. Read lines ()
3. Read line ([n])

At this point, we must surely be wondering what the letter n surrounded in parenthesis and square brackets means. It's pretty simple: the letter n will inform the file of the bytes it will read and analyze.

Read method ([ ])

```
1    myFile = open("D://pythonfile//mypythonfile.txt","r")
2    myFile.read(9)
```

We can see that there is a number 9 inside the read () function, which tells Python that he just needs to read the first nine letters of the file.

Read line Method (n)

```
1    myFile = open("D://pythonfile//mypythonfile.txt","r")
2    myFile.readline()
```

The readline method reads a line from a file and returns the read bytes in the form of a string. Even if the byte n exceeds the line quantity, the readline function can only read one line of code.

It has a syntax that is fairly similar to the read () method.

Readlines Method (n)

The readlines method reads all of the file's lines so that the read bytes can be reassembled into a string. This approach, unlike the readline method, can read all of the lines.

Its syntax is quite similar to that of the read () and readline () methods:

```
1    myfile = open("D:\\pythonfile\\mypythonfile.txt","r")
2    myfile.readlines()
```

After we've opened a file, we can access a variety of
information (attributes) to learn more about it. These
characteristics are:

File.name: The name of the file is returned by this
attribute.

File. Mode: This is an attribute that returns the file
accesses we used to open it.

File. Closed: This is an attribute that returns a "True" if
the file we're working with is closed, and a "False" if the
file we're working with is still open.

Close () function

The close function removes any type of information that
has been written in our program's memory, allowing us
to close the file. However, we can end a file in other ways,
such as when we reassign an object from one file to
another.

The close function has the following syntax:

```
1     myfile.close()
2
```

What exactly is a buffer?

The buffer can be defined as a file that is temporarily stored in ram memory and contains a fragment of data that makes up the sequence of files in our operating system. When working with a file for which the storage size is unknown, we frequently employ buffers.

It's vital to remember that if the file's size exceeds our equipment's ram memory, the processing unit won't be able to run the software and perform its functions appropriately.

What is the purpose of a buffer? The size of a buffer indicates the amount of storage space available while using the file. The application will show us the size of our file in the platform in a specified method using the function: io.DEFAULT BUFFER SIZE.

We can see this more clearly now:

```
1    import io
2        print("Default buffer size:"io.DEFAULT_BUFFER_SIZE)
3        file= open("Myfile.txt", mode= "r", buffering=6)
4        print(file.line_buffering)
5    file_contents=file.buffer
6    for line in file_contents
7        print(line)
```

Errors

We'll look in our files for a string (of the optional type) that specifies how we should handle coding mistakes in our software.

Errors can only be used in text files in the txt form. The following are some of them:

Ignore_errors()	This will avoid the comments with a wrong or unknown format
Strict_errors()	This is going to generate a subclass or UnicodeError in case that any mistake or fail comes out in our code file

Encoding

When working with data storage, we usually utilize string encoding, which is nothing more than a representation of character encoding based on bits and bytes as a representation of the same character.

This is how it's written:

```
1    string.encode(encoding="UTF-8", errors= "strict")
2
```

Newline

The Newline mode is responsible for controlling the functionality of new lines, which can be 'r', " ", none, 'n', and 'rn'.

The newlines are universal and can be thought of as a technique of deciphering our code's text sequences.
1. In Windows, the end-of-line sentence is "rn."

2. Max Os's line-ending sentence: "r."
3. The UNIX end-of-line sentence: "n"

When a newline of type none is entered, the universal newline mode is activated immediately.

Our program automatically converts input lines that finish in "r", "n", or "rn" to "n" before returning them. If their individual legal parameters for coding are met, the lines will be entered just once and their final line will not be translated at the time of return.

On output, any type of character "n" entered will be transformed to a line separator called "os.linesep" if the newline is of the none type.

If the newline is of the type " ", no translator will be created, and if the newline encounters any value that is regarded legal for the code, it will be immediately translated to the string.

For " ", here's an example of newline reading.

```
1    string.encode(mode="r", newline= " ")
2
```

The following is an example of newline reading for none:

```
1    string.encode(mode="w", newline= "none")
2
```

The "os" module allows you to manage your files.

We can use the "os" module to conduct various activities that are dependent on the operating system (actions such as starting a process, listing files in a folder, end process and others).

With the "os" module, we may handle files using a variety of methods, including:

os.makedirs()	This method of the "os" module will create a new file
os.path.getsize()	This method of the "os" module will show the size of a file in bytes.
os.remove(file_name)	This method of the "os" module will delete a file or the program
os.getcwd ()	This method of the "os" module will show us the actual directory from where we will be working
os.listdir()	This method of the "os" module will list all the content of any folder of our file
os.rename (current_new)	This method of the "os" module will rename a file
os.path.isdir()	This method of the "os" module will transfer the parameters of the program to a folder
os.chdir()	This method of the "os" module will change or update the direction of any folder or directory
os.path.isfile()	This method of the "os" module will transform a parameter into a file.

Xlsx files: What exactly are xlsx files? They are spreadsheet-related files. This is essentially the same as dealing with spreadsheet apps like Excel. For example, if we use the Windows operating system on our computer, we can benefit from the fact that working with these types of files is much lighter than working with other types of files.

When working with databases, statistics, calculations, numerical type data, images, and even some sorts of rudimentary automation, xlsx files come in handy.

We will learn how to interact with the basic features of this sort of file in this chapter, which include creating, opening, and changing files.

To get started, we'll need to install the necessary library, which we can accomplish by typing "pip3 install openpyxl" into our Python terminal.

After running this command, the openpyxl module will be downloaded and installed in our Python files. We can also check for documentation to learn more about this module.

Create an xlsx file: Let's use the openpyxl () Workbook () function to create an xlsx file with this module.

```python
from openpyxl import Workbook
def xlsxdoc():
    wb = Workbook()
    sheet = wb.active
    name = "test.xlsx"
    wb.save(name)
xlsxdoc()
```

This is the first step in managing files of the type xlsx; as you can see, we first generated the file by importing the function Workbook from the module openpyxl, and then we assigned the function Workbook to the variable wb () With this, we proclaim that this is the document with which we will be working (we create the object in the form of a worksheet in this format). After that, we activate the object with the name wb, assign it a name, and lastly save the file.

With this module, you may add the following information to the file:

We'll need to use another set of functions available with the object to add information to our file, one of which is the append method.

```
1    from openpvxl import Workbook
2    def xlsxdoc():
3        wb = Workbook()
4        sheet = wb.active
5        sheet = ["B4"] = "Goodnight"
6        name = "test.xlsx"
7        wb.save(name)
8    xlsxdoc()
```

We can see that this is similar to the last example in which we needed to build a document; we followed the same steps: we formed the object wb in the function xlsxdoc (), activated the object, and entered the information there. We'll need to know the exact location where we'll put in this new space; in this case, we'll write "B4" in the fourth box of the second row, and these will be matched with a string that says "goodnight." The last stages are the same as in the previous example, so we'll just type in a name and save it using the save command.

We can write and enter data in a more straightforward manner by using the add function ()

```python
from openpyxl import Workbook
def xlsxdoc():
    wb = Workbook()
    sheet = wb.active
    messages = ("Hello" , "good morning", "goodnight" )
    sheet.append = (messages)
    name = "test.xlsx"
    wb.save(name)
xlsxdoc()
```

We can see that we produced the document "test.xlsx" using the processes we described earlier, and we can also see that we created a tuple called messages, which has three items:

"Hello," "good morning," and "goodnight" are common greetings.

After we've constructed the tuple, we'll use the append method to attach all of the information included in the tuple messages, and then save the document with the save function.

What does it mean that the add () method only accepts iterable data? This refers to data of type arrangements, tuples, because our software will return an error if they are not entered in this manner.

Read documents in xlsx

```python
1    from openpyxl import Workbook
2    name = "test.xlsx"
3    def xlsxdoc():
4        wb = load_Workbook(name)
5        sheet = wb.active
6        file1 = sheet["C1"].value
7        file2 = sheet["C2"].value
8        file3 = sheet["C3"].value
9        print(file1)
10       print(file2)
11       print(file3)
12   xlsxdoc()
```

Returning to our initial example of getting data from xlsx files, we can see that we used the load workbook class for this. The name of the file we want to open is the first thing we need to know, so we established a variable with that name.

It's crucial that the files are in the same folder as the application, or else the software will give us an error. Within the function xlsdoc(), we will create the object wb, which will represent the sheet that we will use, and then the object "sheet," which will represent the sheet that we will use.

After that, we will request information from the specific boxes "C1", "C2", and "C3" adjacent to the function value, and we will publish all of the information asked to ensure that the information we obtain is accurate.

Working with PDF files

The beginnings of this sort of file are known as "Portable Document Format," which have increased in popularity over time and are primarily utilized in business and education. This is due to the fact that they offer a plethora of advantages, like the ability to set access keys to limit who may change the document and even a watermark to prevent material from being plagiarized.

Other noteworthy information is that these documents can be seen on any device because they do not require a specific program; additionally, the file weight is much reduced because the texts are compressed, unlike Word documents.

One downside of PDF files is that they are difficult to alter once they are created.

We will just learn how to produce PDF files in this chapter. To produce a PDF file, we must first download the library using the command "Pip3 install fpdf," after which we may proceed to create our document as follows:

```python
from fpdf import FPDF

pdfdoc = PDF()
pdfdoc.set_font('Times New Roman', 'B', 12)
pdfdoc.add_page()
pdfdoc.cell(12, 10, "First PDF program", 5, 6, "C")
pdfdoc.output("first PDF", 'F')
```

This is a low level example, but it is significantly more complex than other file kinds. To begin a document, we will import the FPDF class from the fpdf library, then create the pdfdoc object, which will be the pdf document. We'll need to adjust the forms, size, and style of the letters we'll be using once we've produced this document. The command set font is used to accomplish this.

Times New Roman will be the font of choice in this scenario, with a bold style and a size of 12.

Following that, we'll use the command add page () to add a page because we'll need one to write on, and the function fpdf doesn't produce a blank page by default. Then we'll use the cell () function, which has a number of crucial arguments, to input information.

The cell function will contain the width and height that the cell will occupy, as well as the message that will be printed in string format. If further detail is necessary on the edges, we must add 1 to the cell function, as the default value of 0 does not allow anything to be put.

If you want to add a cell below or to the right, type 0; otherwise, type 1. A string will be placed if you want the text to be centered to the right, left, up, or down; if you want it to be centered, type C.

Finally, we must save the document using the output () command, with the arguments being the file name (with the ".pdf" inserted because we want a pdf file) and the string "F."

Taking care of BIN files

As we previously discussed, not all files are text files. These can also be handled by lines, and there are some files that, when processed, each byte has a special meaning for the software; as a result, they must be altered in their original format.

The files in Binary are a good example of this; working with these files is as simple as adding a b to the parameter mode's space.

Consider the following scenario:

```
1   with open("pythonfile", "rb") as f:
2       byte = f.read(4)
3       while byte:
4           byte = f.read(4)
```

It's critical to understand the present position of the data we need to edit while working with a binary file. If you don't know where you are in the file, the file. Tell () function will tell you how many bytes have passed since we started it.

We utilize the function file if we wish to change the current position in the file.

Seek (star, from) will allow us to move a set number of bytes from beginning to end.

Conclusion

Thank you for reading all the way to the finish in order to learn Python programming language faster and easier. We hope you found it useful and that you were able to use all of the resources offered to accomplish your goals of learning Python programming language.

After reading this book, you should be able to create a variety of programs for various circumstances. The next stage is to continue practicing as much as possible in order to master Python. While programming, you may believe that some things are impossible to code or that you are not capable of doing so. But that isn't true; all you have to do is think hard enough to make it happen. Also, while programming, you may discover that your code or program does not work; do not be concerned; even the most intelligent people develop code that does not work at first. All you have to do now is keep trying.

As you may be aware, technology and programming are ubiquitous nowadays. We encourage that you try to code and solve problems in your daily activities in order to extend your perspective on the world, as all devices include hundreds of lines of code.